The Average American Son

Trent M. Harris

I0450254

iUniverse, Inc.
New York Lincoln Shanghai

The Average American Son

Copyright © 2005 by Trent M. Harris

iUniverse books may be ordered through booksellers or by contacting:

iUniverse
2021 Pine Lake Road, Suite 100
Lincoln, NE 68512
www.iuniverse.com
1-800-Authors (1-800-288-4677)

ISBN: 0-595-34282-5 (pbk)
ISBN: 0-595-67094-6 (cloth)

Printed in the United States of America

The Average American Son

Contents

Part IV   Self Destruction

Author's Note

I am unable to unspill the water I have spilt during my life. All I can do is clean up the mess and move on. While I was doing this, I came across a story I had written when I was fifteen. *A Murder Story* was published on a limited basis and did not sell well at all, but seeing it, lying in the dusty boxes filled with many other memories of times long since passed, triggered a radical change in my life.

This book I wrote so many years ago recaptured my longing to be writer. Along with *A Murder Story, Awakening, Christopher, The Xebec,* and *Rich Hill* sat collecting dust. To me they represented dreams lost—dreams forgotten before life had its chance to hang itself around my neck, but they became the hope I needed to move forward. From that moldy box of memories, I found something to work towards, something to look forward too.

After rediscovering them, I sat down and read through all of them twice, nearly twelve-hundred pages, covering ten years of my life. Each story took place during a particular part of my life and captured the people around me, the problems and successes of my life, and wrapped everything up in a horrific story line of terror in my home town of Centerburg. It did not take long for the hopes of past dreams to reseed themselves and begin to move my life once again in a positive direction.

I once again set out with a passion to have my stories published. This new drive led to the completion of my college degree, the completion of a master's degree, and has led me into film school. Doors that were once closed have now opened, and each morning is a new adventure into the potential life has to offer.

When it finally came time to republish *A Murder Story* and to prepare the other novels for publication, it was brought to my attention the books had a common thread leading one book into the next. Each take place in Centerburg, Ohio, the plot lines cross, and common characters are used. They are a series that grounds its basis in my own personal experiences growing up in small town America.

Since the characters, the settings, the sub crisis's, and the content are reflections of my experiences, it was decided to write the true story behind these five books. At first I was not interested in writing a true story about my life. In general, life is relatively mundane and routine. Achievements or failures are a small part of ones life. The rest is filled with the repetitiveness of everyday life. I prefer exciting fiction, filled with monsters and ghouls, but took the advice I was given and wrote *The Average American Son* to lay the foundation for *The Centerburg Horrors*, as they are now being called.

I can not write about my entire life, just where I have already been. I broke my life up into chapters, discussing everything I believe to be relevant as I was raised in an average home, in a Midwestern town, with average parents. The early part of the book is written from my parents' perspectives as they saw the truth, but the rest was written through my eyes and reflects my impression of the world and the situations around me.

This is not the most exciting book, but it reflects life which is seldom filled with constant thrill. I left the thrill for *The Centerburg Horrors*, to be released soon after, starting with *A Murder Story*.

A Special Thanks To:

Nick Stockdale
Brandon Roth
Daniel Crews
Ben Scribner
Han Tan

This book was written in the basement of a house in Lynchburg, Virginia, while I was going to college at Liberty University. During my stay there I had the pleasure of having these five people as roommates. They soon became good friends of mine and were extremely supportive during a time when I needed it the most. Though our time together was relatively short, it was an era in my life I will never forget. I will remember each of them for the rest of my life and wish them all the very best in everything they pursue. Their friendship is priceless and will affect everything I do.

PART I
The Beginning

1

Calvin L. Harris

I do not remember much of my early childhood; like many, I have had to put it together from those who were around at the time. I gathered the stories from family members, friends of the family, and put together a picture of what my life was like before the age of three.

I was born in Lynchburg, Virginia, on October 11, 1976 to the parents of Charlotte Harris and Calvin Harris. They had been married for six years before my birth and lived a life of rebellion and complacency. My dad, Calvin, grew up in Appomattox, Virginia, raised by his grandmother. He had two sisters Patricia and Shirley, all three growing up in a life of poverty in the hills of the Blue Ridge.

My dad never really had a stable home life growing up. His father being a severe alcoholic, unable to carry a job and very abusive to his children, and his mother, not having the mental capacity to carry on daily activities, much less raise children, left my dad and his sisters in limbo when it came to were they would sleep, where there meals came from, and who would look out for their well being.

With both parents unable to care for the three children, they were passed from person to person, anyone who would take them and relieve the burden of child rearing from the parents. Often the children were split up. My dad would live with one welcoming person or family while his two sisters lived with someone else.

I recently was able to go back to Appomattox and see first hand one of the places my dad lived. It horrified me! Even in its best day, it was nothing more then a shack with no running water, no electricity, and deep within the pine-woods of the area. The small house was just three rooms, which entailed a dirt floor and open ceiling exposing the underside of the tin roof. I tried to imagine what it was like in the winter with the cold air blowing in though the cracks in the planked walls and the damp dirt floors. It was beyond my comprehension. All my life, I simply had to worry about a cool draft after stepping out of a hot shower or the occasional draft from an unsealed window. I never worried about the cold dirt beneath my feet or wondered whether hot water would warm my bath before I went to bed in a centrally heated home, with the occasional electric blanket on those really cold nights.

I used to think the stories my dad told me about him having to get a job bailing hay to pay for shoes was made up to instill an appreciation for the many things my parents had provided for me. We have all heard the stories about having to walk in the snow two feet deep, up hill both ways to school. Parents have been telling those stories to whining children for years in hopes of showing them how lucking they were to be catching a heated bus or having someone pick them up on those cold days.

I discovered my dad actually did those things. Well, maybe not walk to school in snow two feet deep uphill both ways. Instead, he did not go to school on those snowy days. He chopped wood to keep him and his caretakers just above freezing in their breezy home. He made money to get his shoes by picking up soda bottles along the side of the roads weaving between the tobacco fields. He had to work to go to school. School was a privilege to him and his sisters. It they had the clothing and the chores were done, they were allowed to go school.

This was the childhood life of my father—one filled with hard work, very little guidance, and few who cared about his well being. It was just him up against the world. I could not dream of not having someone to come home to—someone who missed you when you were gone. But my dad did not have this. He was considered a nuisance and a burden to both his parents and to those who had to take care of him. He was considered a mistake and was treated like one. People did all they could to get rid of the mistake, but my dad held in there. He made it through high school and caught his way out of the cruel poverty by enlisting in the US Army.

He enlisted in the Army at a time when the country was knee deep in the Vietnam War and all the horrors of that war. He pulled two tours of duty in the muck of Vietnam and made it through some of the most horrid conditions imaginable.

I do not have a point of reference to describe what my dad went through while he was over seas serving his country, but he did his best to let my brother and I know what he did for this country and what the others serving with him did for this country.

When I was old enough to understand the depictions of war my dad had floating through his mind, he expressed them to me as best he could. He told me about walking through the jungle brush in the pouring rain, soaked to the skin with parasites eating at his flesh. His feet became so raw from the water logged socks, the skin would peal from the heal and ball of his feet.

Sleep was a thing of the past. He survived on cat knaps caught between the chaos of bullet ridden skirmishes hoping the enemy would not sneak up on him as he caught five minutes of rest. So tired were he and his fellow soldiers, they could sleep standing up, leaning against a tree soaked to the bone in pouring rain. Sleep deprivation became a way of life.

He would eat the rations the military provided. Still fine-tuning the art of providing soldiers with food out in brush, most of the rations were spoiled, or filled with worms. The small amounts of Tang his sister sent him would make the river water taste of sweet orange and not the bitter taste of rotting plant and animal life. So prized was a Pepsi, soldiers would spend twenty dollars or more for a single can.

As if the lack of sleep for long periods of time and eating spoiled food was not bad enough, these soldiers had to deal with the horrors of war on a day after day basis. They were left out in the bush for days, with the goal of securing villages, or scouting out enemy positions. They saw first hand the inherent evil of man.

My dad told me tails of walking past trees with women nailed to them, their unborn babies dangling from their lacerated abdomens. He recounted a time when he had to carry his friend out of the bush in his helmet. A mortar had shredded his friend's body, but he was able to collect a foot and hand from the buddy he had vowed to back up in the heat of battle. He didn't have enough time to look for other parts, but he gathered what he could, placed the parts in his helmet and continued into the brush behind enemy lines.

Through hard work and dedication to his country, despite the relentless horror of what he had to do, my dad moved up in rank to Sergeant. He was nineteen, seven years younger then I am right now as I write this book when he received this promotion. He was given a group of privates and sent back into the jungles to continue to fight for Americans a world away.

On his second tour, a bullet grazed the top of his head, and scrap metal was blown into his lower back by a rouge grenade. He told me his near misses with death did not disturb him as much as entering villages. At this point in the war, the warfare of the enemy had changed. On his first tour, intelligence told him where the enemies were lying wait and the battles were between solders. On his second tour, civilians started to play in the enemy's battle plan.

Before, he would enter a village and the people of the village would welcome their presence and their protection, but that had changed. Now the enemy would strap live grenades to the backs of children, some as young as six, and have them walk up to the approaching soldiers. While the soldier was reassuring the child everything would be all right, the grenades would detonate, and the child would rip in two along with the comforting soldier. Pieces of the child would spatter the other soldiers while their comrade lay shredded at their feet.

This would happen many times before my dad and his soldiers simply had no other choice but to shoot anyone who approached them. Before they did everything to protect the women and children, now they were forced to execute anyone who came near them.

For a while no one approached the troops as they secured the villages. The villagers knew the American soldiers had been attacked in this way and were protecting themselves. They respected the distance required by the troops.

Again, the enemy's tactics changed. The adversary would hold a child's mother or father at gun point or vise versa and make that person run towards the approaching troops. Sometimes the children would get through and obliterate themselves and a couple troops, often times the soldiers were forced to kill the innocent running towards them.

My dad spoke of this repeatedly throughout his life. I am sure there were times he killed a young man or woman only to get to the bloodied body to see they were unarmed. Killing a child who turned out to have explosives strapped to their back would have been bad, but to kill a child who was just happy to see relief come their way would have been devastating to a soldier.

With these horrors behind him, my dad came home; back to Virginia. He was proud of his military accomplishments. He was not proud of the killing, but he was proud he had served his country. He had pulled himself out of extreme poverty and served his fellow Americans in an honorable manner.

He had saved the small paychecks the Army had given him and bought a piece of land and a new car when he got back to The States. He came back to America with such great expectations. He had suffered his childhood in scarcity, with no one to care for him, and had endured two horrific tours of duty in Vietnam. He was looking forward to a new start. He had a small piece of land in his home state of Virginia and had a car that became his pride and joy. But what he came home to was not what he had imagined.

He returned to an America that hated him. He had killed for America and would have died for America. He brought back the remains of his friends who had died for America, and the people walking down the streets spit on his uniform. He constantly had to wipe the phlegm from his medals of honors. The uniform he had worked so hard to be able to come home in was now a symbol of hatred. They looked at him as if he was a Nazi as he walked down the streets of his hometown.

Just a few days after returning, the people he had sworn to protect had destroyed his hopes of heroism. He folded his uniform and placed in a trunk at the foot of his bed and placed his metals into a cigar box. He was forced to hide the blood he had shed for his country. In my Dad's eyes, he was failure. He was just a poor country boy who no loved or even cared if he returned from war.

Eventually, the horrors of war started to way on him, but he stood strong for several years. He went to work and became a productive member of society. Just like he had in his past, he stood strong. In this strength he met my mother and they fell in love.

2

Charlotte H. Wills

In my recount of my mother's life, I am going to lean heavily on her perspective of her childhood. Just like I did with my dad, I want to capture the essence of what she held of value growing up and how she saw her youth when she looked back. I am sure there will be some errors in my recount of her childhood, but the following is a narration as she saw it. Her perspective on her childhood had a great deal in shaping the woman she became. Whether she interpreted her past correctly or accurately is irrelevant.

It is evident my mother grew up differently than my father. She came from a loving family in the heart of Campbell County, Virginia. On March 24, 1949, my mother was born. Her mother, Gladys, named her Charlotte Hope Wills. She was Gladys's second child. Her older sister Doris had been born a couple years earlier and was followed by her younger sister Wanda.

Sometime when all three children were very young, Gladys separated from her husband William and remarried Randolph, who I would later know as Pa-Pa. The three children grew up with Randolph as their father. They did not find out he wasn't their biological father until much later in their lives.

All three referred to Randolph as Daddy, and he took up the roll very well. There is much to be said about this man. He married Gladys at a time when divorce was not commonplace and took up the fatherhood role of three girls that were not even his. He was a very admirable man, and that admiration can be seen and reflected in the love of the three children he raised.

When my mother spoke of her step-dad, she often referred to a fond memory that clearly showed the dedication her daddy had to the well being of his wife's daughters. My mother came down with Scarlet Fever as a young child. At the time this was a serious ailment, often fatal in the young and old. She was running extremely high fevers, unable to keep anything on her stomach, and was in flu like agony that concerned her parents deeply.

Late into the night, with her dad sitting beside her bed keeping a cold rag on her head to help with the fever, my mother made a request. She asked for some grape juice. That was all she wanted. Her body was dehydrated, and she wanted some fresh juice to quench her thirst.

Randolph, clearing the sleep from his head was ecstatic with her request. After several days of vomiting and sweating profusely from fever, his little girl wanted something to drink. Her stomach had settled enough for juice.

He gladly put on his cloths and set out to fulfill the request of his precious, still high on the notion she was getting better and that the worse was over. With Gladys left at my mother's bedside, Randolph went out into the night to get grape juice. She had made a request and the adventure began for him—an adventure only a loving parent would endure for simply a smile from his sick daughter.

When I look at this story from my life in today's society, I am at a loss as to what my grandfather went through to get this grape juice for my mother. Today I would be able to get anything I needed pretty much at anytime I needed it. If I want some grape juice, it would be a ten-minute ordeal to the local grocery no matter what time of day I needed the beverage. But my grandfather was up against the times in which he lived. There were no twenty-four hour convenience stores or groceries to go to, especially in the small community in which he lived. He had a real challenge to find something so simple.

Of course he took on that challenge full force. His daughter had asked her knight in shining armor to bring her some juice, and he was going to fulfill her request. He drove from store to store looking for that one that would be open at such a late hour. All the while he was driving through the night, his mind raced of the fantastic turn of events in his daughter's health.

After checking all the stores in his local community, he drove to other cities looking for grape juice. He would not stop until he found what he needed and returned home. City after city, store after store, he came up empty handed. There did not seem to be a place open in the entire world that could help him out that night. But, he drove on.

After several hours of checking every place he could find, my grandfather found a small convenience store open all night. He rushed in, found the juice he needed and headed home. He had waged through the urges to sleep and found his daughter's grape juice.

He drove home with a sense of pride for his accomplishment. He was going to be able to provide his daughter with her heart's desire that night. This elation swept away the weariness from the lack of sleep, the frustration of going to so many places, and he was filled with the joy only a father can of being able to provide for his ailing child.

It took him a while to get home after driving so far away, but he did not waste any time when he pulled into the driveway. He got out of his car and rushed into the house with the juice. Being quiet not to wake his other daughters, he quickly poured some of the ever so valuable juice into a glass and went straight to my mother's room.

I am not sure if Gladys was in my mother's room sleeping when my grandfather came back or if she had went back to the comfort of her own bed. I do know my mother was sound asleep. Her fever had broken, and she was finally able to rest. It was the best sleep she had been able to get since being sick. Her color was turning to normal, and the constant flu pains that had plagued her had let up.

After pouring a generous helping of the grape elixir, my grandfather entered my mother's room. He was so proud of his accomplishment; he did not notice how peacefully she was sleeping. He gently nudged her shoulder with the anticipation of his daughter's joy at the sight of the grape juice.

My mother, deep in her needed sleep, groggily turned over in her bed to look at her daddy. There he stood with the juice he spent most the night looking for, smiling from ear to ear.

"Here baby, I have your grape juice," he said, gently placing the glass within her reach.

Annoyed at being awakened from her needed slumber, my mother answered, "Grape juice? Daddy, I don't want grape juice anymore. I just want to go back to sleep."

With a single motion, my mother pulled the covers over her shoulders and quickly drifted back into the comfort of her painless sleep. My grandfather, still smiling, placed the glass of juice on the nightstand and tucked his daughter in for the night. He was not disappointed his beloved daughter no longer wanted the juice. He saw she was better and sleeping comfortable, and that was enough for him.

With the all night drive completely forgotten, my grandfather went to bed knowing his daughter would be fine. The weight of a sick child had been lifted from his shoulders, and now he could sleep. My mother had not been the only person in the house not sleeping. He was sleepless with his daughter, but his love for her overcame the sleepless nights, the constant worry, and the all night drive. He was content with her sleeping soundly in her bed that night.

This was just one of many instances where my grandfather demonstrated his love for my mother and her sisters while they were growing up. He took on a role that is hard to do, even in today's more understanding society with all the conveniences the last twenty years have brought.

A story comes to mind when I think about my time in high school and the constant push my mother had for me to do well in school. She was like most mother's when it came to her children doing well in school, but my mother had a background of doing poorly in school until an event occurred causing her to become an exceptional student.

When she was in grade school, she played kick ball every moment of the day regardless of the consequences. I am sure her parents were on her to do her homework, study for her tests, and to listen in class, but like most children, school was not the most important thing in her life. Kick ball was. She had a love for sports at a very young age; something that she would excel at in high school, but in grade school caused her many problems.

As time went by, the school tests were failed and homework was not turned in. She went through several pairs of shoes during that time, placing a burden on her parents to replace the worn soled shoes she seemed to go through on a monthly basis. Her family was just a middle class family and did not have the money to replace shoes every couple of months. They relied on hand-me-downs to stretch money, but with her going through so many shoes, there was nothing to hand down to her younger sister, and her older sister was not going through them at the rate she was.

Her mother and father did what they could to keep shoes on her feet, but my mother continued to wear them out spending her time playing kick ball at school and with the local children in her neighborhood. But, the days of carefree kickball at the park came to quick end at the end of that school year.

The school my mother was attending felt it would be necessary to hold her back a year due to her poor performance. They did not feel she was at an educational disadvantage; it was just that she was not applying herself. She didn't do her homework or study or listen in class; instead, she planned her next game at the local park or at recess.

When all of us look back, most of us can recount a moment in our youth when certain realities of the world became very clear to us. This was one of those moments for her. She had a very basic understanding of what the consequences of not studying or doing homework meant in her school life.

They held her back for a year. She had to watch all her friends move on to the next grade while she was repeating the year. She often spoke of this and how humiliating it was to her. She had to explain to her friends she had not passed;

she had to explain to a new class of students as to why she did not move on, and she had to make all new friends.

This humiliation was a driving force in her young life. She devoted herself from that point on to doing well in school. She studied constantly and did her homework. This new motivating force in her life stayed with her throughout even high school. She did not want to have to go through failure again.

As I look at her life, I can point to this instance as to when my mother decided she would give her all too every task she did. Other life experiences shaped her work ethic and frugalness, but this seems to be the beginning of her work hard and long mentality.

This memory of humiliation carried over into her parenting skills with my brother and I. She was consistently on us about doing our schoolwork before we did anything else. She did not want us to have to go through what she did when she played kickball instead of doing her schoolwork.

The rest of her preteen life was very similar to that of any other southern family at the time. She went to church with her sisters on Sunday, school during the week. She had daily chores to help around the house since both her mother and father worked to keep the roof over their heads and food in their bellies.

On Saturdays, she cleaned house from top to bottom, staring early in the morning, having the afternoons open to play with her sisters or do her homework from the previous week. This became the norm for my mother; her life was filled with the routines of daily life as she grew into a young woman.

My mother was also a fire child when she was young, like me. It is one of the things the two of us shared in common in our young age. We both liked to play with fire. I was caught numerous times catching my G. I Joes on fire or playing with fire crackers, and she did the same in her youth.

She liked to take toilet paper and run it down the driveway and light it on fire watching it burn in its fiery strip. When she was caught, she was dealt with severely. Her parents were petrified that she would burn the house down, or even worse, hurt herself playing with the fascinating flames.

In time, just like me, she grew out of the fire fascination. I am not sure if she stopped because she out grew it or if she stopped for the reason I stopped. I was tired of being grounded and spanked for playing with the flames. In any case, she stopped, but remembered her experience with fire when she dealt with me twenty years later.

She made it through grade school and middle school doing very well academically and started getting back into her passion for sports. She picked up basketball in high school and excelled. She received her letter from Brookville High to put on her school sweater or jacket and took home numerous trophies for her athletic ability.

She did well in high school. She was successful in basketball and did well in her classes. From my understanding she was also very popular and had many friends; but the humiliation of her grade school failure kept her at home and studying at night instead of going out with her friends to have a good time. She went to school and basketball but did very little with the people at her school outside of school activities.

She graduated from high school at the head of her class and went out into the work force to start building her life as an adult. It is uncertain as to what happened during the time from her graduation to her meeting my father, but I think she was doing many of the things any young person would do.

My mother grew up in a household filled with love and understanding unlike the childhood life of my father. Both came from very different backgrounds, but they came together and fell in love.

3

Mr. And Mrs. Calvin Harris

The beginnings of my parent's relationship are very sketchy; I just have bits and pieces of it to incorporate into this story. But the points I have, carried over into my life as a young child and into my young adult life.

My parents met through my mother's younger sister Wanda. She was dating my father's cousin E.G. and my dad and him were good friends. As Wanda brought E.G. around, my dad started to come into the picture. The four of them did things together, and those outings started the initial relationship between my mother and father.

From talking with my mom's sisters, I have a picture of my mom at the time when my dad started to come around. My mother had very poor self-esteem when it came to the men in her life. There really were no boyfriends in the past or any other men who tried to fill the position for my mother.

In listening to my mother's recounts of her high school life, there were no fellows around and if there were, she simply pushed them away because of her own insecurities. Sometimes people will push others away when they feel they are not worthy of their companionship, and I believe this was one reason my mother did not date. I think there were boys asking her out when she was in high school, but she said no or didn't give them the opportunity to ask.

When my dad came around, she was not spending time with him directly but spending time with her sister and her boyfriend, my dad just happened to be there. Just like today, if you put two young people together for a long enough period of time, things are going to start to happen, especially if both are single and looking for some sort of a relationship. This is how it began between my parents.

My mother saw a man who was showing her the attention she felt she had never received from a man before. She saw my dad as the first man who looked at her in a romantic way and gave her the attention she so longed for from a man.

Just coming out of the military after serving in Vietnam, my dad was in his prime when it came to his looks and his outlook on life.

After going out with her sister and boyfriend, my mother and father starting dating on their own. They started to develop the relationship between them. What started out as convenience dates to fill the gaps when hanging out with Wanda and E.G. blossomed into a steady relationship between my mom and dad.

It is interesting to note my dad did not have a driver's license when they first starting dating. After getting back from Vietnam my dad used his money to purchase a 1965 Chevy Malabo and had supercharged it to run far faster then it should have on public roads. He was caught many times drag racing through the streets of Lynchburg, Virginia, and finally, after a police chase, the judge pulled his license.

He was a hellcat on the open road and lost his privilege to drive for a year. E.G. was his closest friend and designated driver while he was under suspension. Because of this my dad had to tag along when he went to visit his girlfriend, bringing my dad in contact with my mother.

It is interesting to see how seemingly chance occurrences bring two people together—two people who had little in common and very different backgrounds.

Time went by and the relationship matured to a point where marriage came into focus. They had dated for a while and both were now ready to take the next step. Even with the many differences between the two, they still decided it was time to begin their lives together.

When my dad purposed to my mother, he left here a watch on her car seat. By this time, she was the one doing all the driving, and it was a certainty she would find the gift. I can remember this watch throughout my childhood. My mother wore it as a reminder of the love they had shared.

Sometime during this courting between my parents, differences started to creep into my mother's relationship with her parents. I am not sure if my grandfather disapproved of the marriage, but I am certain my grandmother did.

The wedding was held without the attendance of my mother's parents. They simply sent an ironing board as a wedding present and put the matter behind them. My mom never fully forgave her parents for this. She always remembered how her mom and dad were not at the wedding.

I am not completely positive as to what caused the drift in my mother's relationship with her parents, but it is apparent it came to a head with the marriage. They never accepted the marriage and did very little to help support the newly wed couple. This gap would not be fully bridged until I was born many years later.

My parents started out with very little, like most newly wed couples. After returning from their honeymoon at Williamsburg, Virginia, they rented an attic apartment in Lynchburg. They lived above an elderly woman who was constantly hot regardless of the temperature outside. My dad would have to run the shower with the bathroom door open to allow the steam to warm the one room attic apartment. It wasn't that they could not afford the heat; they simply could not turn it on. The thermostat was located in the main part of the house. Since the woman living in that part was perpetually hot, the heat was never turned up enough to heat the attic. But that did not matter to them. They were together and that was all that mattered at the time. My dad eventually got his license back and let up on the lead foot, learning his lesson after walking for a year. My mom worked odd jobs until she finally got on at Nationwide Insurance.

With both of them working and the lack of children, they were able to buy their first home. It was simple, but it was enough for them to get started. They put a lot of TLC into their new home, fixing all the leaks in the roof, weather proofing the drafty windows, and touching up the faded paint; but it was theirs, and symbolized the official start of their lives together.

My dad did various things to make money. He worked at the Lynchburg Foundry and was going to school at the local community college to become a radiology technician, but he found his love in auto body repair. He had the artistic gift needed to paint cars and scenes on customized vans—so popular at the time. He was able to air brush any scene he wanted on the side of a van, the fuel tank of a motorcycle, or even the motorcycle helmet, often to match the fuel tank.

What once started as a hobby became his obsession. He brought home wrecked car after wrecked car, to fix the bodywork and resell them. He also began restoring old cars he would take to shows and to use as proof of his artistic gift.

My mother settled in at Nationwide and became a productive member of its mailroom, working hard to save her money so her and her husband could purchase another house in a better neighborhood. They wanted to move up, so to speak.

With both working together to move forward, they soon were able to purchase a new home on Newberne Street in Lynchburg, just a stones through from Lynchburg College, and just down the street from Thomas Road Baptist Church. This would be the home that would see the birth of both my brother and I.

This new home of theirs had a lasting impact on their lives. All throughout my life when we would come back to Lynchburg to visit, we would always stop at the old house on Newberne to visit with the friends they had made during my parents stay on that street.

This was the first house that became a home to my parents and to my brother and me. We were a part of that community and settled in with the comfort of the friends of the neighborhood. Many of the people there when we lived there are still there today. The house is still there and still looks as it does in the old pictures I dug out in the family photo album.

They created the perfect place to start a family. They even got a little dog to scurry around the house. It was a black poodle they named Noisy, and as her name implies she was very noisy and into everything. Even though this dog was a poodle it was not treated like a poodle with the puffballs of hair with a prissy personality. My parents kept her hair cut but let the dog be a dog.

Noisy was allowed to dig in the backyard and became the fearless defender of the house. She would even bring the occasional present to my parents and leave them on their bed like any grateful dog would.

I can even recall an instance when Noisy brought my parents a dead chicken and placed in their bed. I guess she wanted to make sure everyone got something to eat that night, but my mother did not see the effort that went into the gift. She just wanted the dead chicken out of her bed. I don't think anyone actually knew where she got the chicken, but it was the only time Noisy brought one to them; so I guess either the owner of the chicken had just one chicken or put up a better fence to keep the dogs out.

After that, it was just the occasional dead mouse or piece of trash rooted out of the neighbor's trash left as gifts. This was obviously before the strict leash laws of today, but no one in the neighborhood seemed to mind. I am sure the neighbors' dogs were roaming the neighborhood with Noisy, having their doggie adventures in a time before dogs would be chained to dog houses or metal stakes in the ground.

My two parents had settled into their lives as husband and wife and had become a part of the community in which they lived. They had started out bumpy without the blessing of my mother's parents but had achieved a degree of success. Starting out in a one-room apartment, moving into a small fixer home, they now entered into a community of modest but comfortable homes and settled into their new lives together.

In looking back, I can honestly say this was the best time the two of them would have together. They were happy and in love and that seemed to blind them from the problems that began to creep into their lives.

4

Directions Change

When people ignore problems in their lives or the potential for problems, life has a way of forcing a solution to those problems. Sometimes issues come to a head demanding to be addressed in a very apparent way. Other times, problems build until there is nothing left but radical corrective action, often times destroying the lives of those involved. This would be the case for my parents.

Being married at an early age, in their early twenties, my parents began to go through growth and maturity changes. What worked at the beginning of their marriage was starting to become issues just a few years into their marital bliss.

My dad had married my mother after returning from the Vietnam War. They did not have a relationship or even know each other before his service, but it was becoming apparent the man she married was changing. Like everyone who served in that war, no one was the same when they returned home. It is also obvious these men of service changed again once returning home, often for the worse.

Injuries from the war had caused my dad to start treatment at the veteran's hospital in Salem, Virginia. At first this was a positive thing in his life. He was out working and going to school, doing the best he could with the pains in his back. Scrap metal from a rouge grenade had blasted pieces of metal into his lower and middle back close to his spinal cord. Surgery was not an option due to how close the shards of metal were to his spinal cord. The risk of paralyzsasion was too great to consider surgery. He simply endued the pain, soothing it over with the drugs his doctor prescribed.

He was also getting into his hobby of auto body repair. It actually started to turn into an out of control obsession. He brought many cars home with the dream of fixing them and making a profit. Parts of cars even began working their way from the back yard into the house, to the reproach of his wife.

This obsession of his got in the way of his school. He started to ditch class to work on his dream of rebuilding cars. The auto parts in the backyard gave him an excuse to miss class. Those run down cars were not going to fix themselves. He was the one in charge of doing that.

School had never been his strong point anyway. It did not take much to distract him from his studies. To him, anything was better than sitting in a class and struggling through the work assigned to him. He was not a stupid man; he simply did not like what he was studying. Had he been in an auto shop class, he may have been more enthusiastic about attending class. I am not even sure why he chose radiology. It could have been the influence of my mother who saw auto repair as inferior to other studies.

The pain medication he was taking was also a contributing factor to his lack of drive to complete school. The medications made it difficult to do anything but rest while the drugs took their effect. They wore him out. He started sleeping more, later in the day, and simply did not get up to go to school. This eventually began to take effect on his work habits. He was missing more time from work and started to move from job to job to fill in the gaps when his auto body repair was lacking.

Sleeping later and later into the day, my dad started staying up later and later at night. He began to run the roads at night with friends and associates who were not the best influences.

All of this started happening the same time my mother was changing. Both were starting to move in two very different directions. The dreams they had once shared started moving in two different directions.

Working at Nationwide started to give my mother confidence. She began to develop a personality that demanded a strong work ethic and a positive movement to achieve financial freedom. The class of people my mother started to associate with at work were ladies of refinement and education. These ladies were also very strong willed women who took control of their lives in every respect. This naturally carried over to my mother's life at home.

She turned from a mild manner woman who let the world go by without much effort, to a woman who sought control of every aspect of her daily life. The first to experience this new found confidence was my dad. He was not holding up his part of the deal. He was sleeping all day, not working the way he should, and his studies at school were declining. She had become a take-charge woman and expected the same from her husband.

With this newfound assurance, she began to see herself as better then those around her. My father was having trouble with his war experience and was sliding into a lifestyle that did not compliment her own. This was the beginning of the tensions that slowly crept into their marriage. She did not know how to deal with my father. She could see he was having problems, was a different man than what she married, but she did not know how to cope with his issues.

My dad was once a man who prided himself on dressing in fine clothing, maintaining a high level of grooming, and worked hard to succeed. This was fading week by week. He was not maintaining himself like he should have, and he was not putting in the effort needed to make the marriage work.

My mom would come home to him on the couch with the pill bottles lining the coffee table. He began to waste his life away, and the avenues he did pursue for success were nothing more than dreams that would never come true. The car parts in the backyard started to pile up, and some even found their way into the house they so prided themselves on. Grease and dirt began working its way into the carpeting and on the new furniture. Steady work had become a thing of the past for my father, the void being filled with good intentions but no action.

The roles had changed in my early family. My mother started out as the timid one with my father at the head of the house. Now she was leading the household with my father trailing behind. This role change caused changes in the marriage, an imbalance.

My mother began to resent the man my father had become. My father felt my mother did not understand what he was going through. He lived with the horrors of the Vietnam War, and she could never understand the turmoil he went through, not with the pain in his back, but with the rough memories floating in his head.

Everyday my mother came home to him sleeping or cleaning some random car part in her living room, she began to resent him more and more. He even resented her for the success she was having. This bile eventually led to arguments, and the unraveling of the marriage they had together.

Neither one really understood what the other was going through. My dad was trying to deal with his war experience and was falling into a pit of self-pity and remorse, and my mother was trying to build her professional career and the home life she felt she deserved.

Arguments became more and more frequent, but the two constantly attempted to rekindle the marriage and keep it going. My mother tried to encourage my father and my dad tried to be more understanding of my mother's desire to succeed. But as time went on, it became more and more evident the marriage would not work. The differences were growing, and the gaps were becoming wider.

This was harder on my mother than on my father. Her marriage started out with people saying it would not succeed. Her own mother did not even show up for the wedding as a protest to the union. Now it started to look like it was going to fall apart just like she had been told.

This fear of failure in front of her critics was overpowering. She was determined not to let the projections of those opposing her marriage see her fail. She began working to become more accommodating to the whims of my father, setting aside her pride and putting her efforts into the marriage without the support of her husband.

She was determined not to fail no matter what it took. She lowered her standards to make my father happy while internally resenting the person she was becoming simply to maintain a marriage that was never meant to be.

5

A Child Bridges the Gap

It is often thought a child would help mend differences between a husband and wife. This notion has been around for a while but has been proven to be an ineffective way to save a marriage. Having a child never changes the differences between two people; it simply puts them on hold, festering just beneath the surface.

I am not sure what the atmosphere was like when my mother became pregnant for the first time. Depending to whom I talk with, I received many different versions, but in each of the recounts of this pregnancy one thing seemed to be evident. This was not something wanted by both of my parents. To listen to my mother, she wanted the unborn child as something to look forward to. My father saw it as a chain to a woman and marriage he was no longer interested in.

My mom knew my dad did not want this child; she even confided to me he had told her so. This was something beyond comprehension to her. She had lowered herself to make the marriage work and had become pregnant by a man who was no longer in love with her. She could not understand how he could not want her as a wife and a soon to be mother.

Her heart was broken completely. That heartbreak led to a miscarriage of the child. Her disappointment in her life and her husband led to a miscarriage. When her body let her know something was wrong by continuous bleeding, she tried to get in touch with my father, but he could not be reached. For once in a long time, he was not passed out on the couch or in the yard working on a worn out car.

She eventually miscarried the fetus and flushed it down the toilet. Her soul retched from her. She had flushed a portion of herself down the toilet that day and her outlook on life was bleak at best. She went to the doctor later that day, but they found nothing wrong with her. She had lost her child due to a broken heart.

I do not know where my dad was; only that he could not be reached. I am sure he was relieved when he heard the news. He did not want the child to begin with, and his desires had been given to him.

Even with this tremendous set back, my mother did not give up on her husband; she was determined to make her marriage work. Failure was not an option. She simply buried the traumatic emotions of the loss and went on with her life. She could not let others see how much she hurt or how unhappy she was, especially my father. She dove into her career, and my dad continued his downward spiral. The less contact they had with each other, the better off they were.

Things did eventually start to get better. The time apart during the day seemed to help prevent the arguments. My dad even started to get himself involved in painting cars. He had long ago dropped out of school, but he finally started showing potential in auto body repair and started bringing good steady money into the house.

Life started to get better between the two. It would seem Dad's success doing bodywork had given him a new vigor for life. He did not spend as much time sleeping or running the roads at night. He was pulling himself out of the rut. My mother was doing well at work, and with time and the new enthusiasm of my father; she began to forget about her miscarriage. Time was beginning to mend the emotional scars both of them had suffered. A new start was beginning between the two.

It was not long before my mother became pregnant again. This time, both my mother and father were looking forward to the new baby. They were able to share in the joy of the new child and the family it would create. They both had something to mutually look forward to and to plan for. It was such a radical change between the two. I can only speculate, my father was feeling much better about himself and that self-confidence was carrying over to his marriage. I am convinced my mother was doing all she could to maintain this new found insurgence in her life and was relishing the turn her marriage had taken.

What once looked like a marriage doomed to end, was now on the rise again. Things were getting back to where they need to be. Their dreams and personalities seemed be realigned to one another, and their lives were again moving in concurrent directions. This child, in conjunction with my mother's business success and my father's success in auto body repair, gave them a rallying point they could both agree on.

On October 11, 1976, I was born at Virginia Baptist Hospital in Lynchburg, Virginia. My parents named me Christopher Lee Harris, and together we all started the journey of family life.

I was born several years after the marriage of my parents. They had been through many ups and downs, but it seemed I would bring a new start to their lives and their relationship with their friends and families.

They took me home and put me in my bassinet with a renewed vigor in their lives. The differences that were once pushing them apart were bridged by the birth of their first son. The dream of a successful marriage seemed to be coming true with this life-changing event for them.

6

I Am Given a Brother

After my birth, my parents experienced for a second time a period when their marriage was going well; they were doing well in their careers, and my mother's family was back in her life in a way it had not been before.

She had contact with her family on a regular basis, but the relationship with her mother had never been the same since she married my father. The resentment for the act always seemed to be just under the surface. I was the first boy born by one of Gladys's daughters. I also held the title of the youngest until my brother came along. Both Wanda and Doris had three beautiful daughters she adored, but the sight of her first grandson put a sparkle in her eyes.

I do not have any memory of my grandmother on my mother's side of the family. She died within the first two years of my life; I simply have a few worn photographs to commemorate her life.

My mom often spoke about her mother and the last day she saw her. She remembered her mom was able to feed me ice cream and talked to all of her children before having the massive heart attack. Gladys had been given the opportunity to see all of those she loved before she died, something most do not have the blessing of being able to do.

Often when my mom looked back, she remembered that afternoon before her mother passed away. Those moments were burned into her mind with sharp clarity many years after her death, and she was thankful she had them along with all the others. That day, though very tragic in the loss, was also a day to remember how great her mother, my grandmother, was for her love of life and of her three daughters. Later, the void left by the death of my grandmother would be filled by another woman who became known to me as Jo-Jo. She would fill the place of grandma quite well.

To cope with the loss of her mother, my mom dove herself into work and into ensuring I was a happy baby. She also attached herself more so to my father than to anything else. That was what her husband was for. She had lost the stability of her mother's presence and tried to fill that void with the companionship of my dad.

Time moved on, as it always does, and the loss of her mother started to fade in my mother's memory. Time began to mend the pain of the loss and life went on. It was not long before my mother became pregnant with my brother. This pregnancy was different from mine. I was the child who brought the two of them together. I was the attempt to bring something into my parents' lives that would help cement their failing marriage. My brother was a result of the love for one another.

He was conceived through the continued love my parents had for me and for each other, but this utopia of marriage life would not last long. During my brother's pregnancy, my mother and father started to fall into their old ways, and the problems that almost destroyed their marriage before I was born, started to seep back into their lives.

My mother began to dedicate herself more intently to her work and again to put pressure on my father to do well, to be consistent with his work and ensure he was pursuing a life healthy to the well being of two children. My father began to fall into his old patterns of sleeping in late and roaming the roads at night. He did maintain his love of cars and to body repair of those cars, but his work habits began to affect the work he was able to get and maintain.

My mother saw this in him as her stomach swelled with child. She saw the old ways beginning to take their hold on my father's life, and she was afraid of the path he was leading. To her, it seemed the novelty of having a child would not be enough to keep the two of them together.

I know the marriage began to break up during my brother's pregnancy, but I am unsure who saw the signs first. My dad sunk into his former lifestyle of taking heavy medication and sleeping late into the day, while my mother dedicated her time to her work.

The two of them began to drift. My unborn brother would not be able to bring them back together this time. My birth was an attempt at gluing the marriage together with the prospects of being parents. My brother was the result of the two coming together.

On July 7th, 1978, my brother, David Wayne Harris, was born at Virginia Baptist Hospital in Lynchburg. By the time of his birth my parents had drifted so far apart it was inevitable they would be walking down the path of divorce soon.

In the time between my birth and my brother's, my mother had lost her mother, had been able to put her marriage back together on a temporary basis, and she had successfully started her career at Nationwide Insurance. My father had refined his skills at auto body repair and was able to hold down a job tempo-rarily. But it was not long after David was born that the veil that hid their marital problems was removed. The issues in their lives they had hidden with my birth festered and broke free after David's birth. They no longer could ignore the prob-lems in their lives or pretend they did not exist.

7

A Marriage Falls Apart

The neighbors living next door to my family on Newbern Street became friends with my parents. They were a young couple and had many things in common with one another, so it was natural a friendship would begin to develop.

Flemming and Tommy had settled into their home just as my parents had a few years prior. This young couple living next to us would become a catalyst that would lead to a broken home and a family divided.

After David's birth, my dad began to take the pain killers the veterans' hospital gave to him for the pains in his back. These medications led to problems with maintaining steady work. My dad could not work if he slept till noon and ran the roads at night. He again began to become overly obsessed with the restoration of old cars to sell for a profit. He had worked with many body shop owners who were quite successful at restoring cars or repairing damaged vehicles for customers. My dad had developed a tremendous talent for painting vehicles, whether they were high end paint jobs for one-hundred thousand dollar vehicles or quick paint jobs for a beater vehicle a teenager had bought as their first ride.

For whatever reason, whether it was the drugs, his inherent propensity to do nothing without a push, my dad just dreamed of the success he would have repairing vehicles. He had the skills and the artistic gift to succeed, but his dream never left the dream phase. He would constantly bring home cars and park them in the back yard, always seeing the possible potential for each vehicle but never following through with the repairs. Pieces of vehicles could be found throughout the basement and deep in the backyard, weeds growing through them as they sat never to be used.

My mother saw this and knew the signs. She had worked hard to break the patterns he had set early in their marriage. She gently pushed him to work, to keep decent hours, and to work hard to keep their home and yard in order. Her encouraging shoves were no longer working. The more she pushed the harder he pushed back.

The neighbors who had become friends of the family began to encourage my father to pursue his dreams of fixing old cars. Flemming, with her southern charm, gave my father a listening ear when my mother pushed him to go to work, to get off the pain killers, and stop roaming the roads at night getting into trouble

I can not be sure when the words of encouragement from Flemming started to become a relationship between her and my father. I do know my mother was working hard during the day while they two of them were developing their love affair with one another. This was happening while Flemming's husband Tommy was at work and my mother was at work.

This went on for a while, and the tensions between my mother and father grew exponentially. The resentment my father had towards my mother due to her success at Nationwide ate at him, and my mother's disappointment towards my dad grew every day she came home to him still in bed or out back piling more useless car parts in the yard.

Often my mother had suspicions this affair went on before the birth of my brother. She had been given certain clues when she would come home early for work, but she overlooked these indications of her wondering husband. She focused herself on me and her unborn child. After David was born, things became more evident the affair was happening, but she had no solid proof.

Her gentle pushing became shoves at my father, and the friendship of the neighbor became a safe haven for Dad from a nagging wife. Instead of confronting the problem directly, both of my parents did things to each other to hurt one another for the sole purpose of getting away from each other. My mother would submerge herself in work, and my father would go over to the neighbor's house.

Not long after David was born my mother had to let her husband go. The affair between him and the neighbor was obvious to everyone around her, but she had overlooking the problems with the hope they would go away. She could not admit the marriage she had so desperately wanted was not working just as her parents had predicted. Her pride was on the line, and her self-esteem was crushed as she watched the man she loved move towards the comforts of another woman. The betrayal of trust eventually built to resentment, and my mother left my father.

She took a step many women did not initiate in the late seventies. Unlike today, women did not usually divorce their husbands. The trend for the men to leave their wives was prevalent, but it did not often happen the other way around.

With her two children, my mother left the man she had married, and sought out to start a new life. Her spirit was broken emotionally and she would have to make drastic changes in her life in order to regain herself emotionally and rebuild her self worth.

My dad had crushed her, but she started to rebuild immediately after leaving the house they had purchased and remodeled. At first she saw her life ending, but this was the beginning of a truly successful life filled with her two sons, many dear friends, and financial and professional success.

8

A Divorce from the Old

Her spirits had been broken and her bullheaded belief that she knew what was best for her had led her to a divorce from the man her parents warned her would never work. Her parents even protested by not showing up for the wedding. Now my mother had to face these failures. She had to look at those who had told her it would not work out and concede to them. They had been right, and she was now paying the consequences of her actions.

She took David and me and tried to restart her life with just the three of us against the world. Instead of becoming humble and accepting her failures and moving on with her life, she filled herself with the determination not to let this happen to her again and to prove to everyone around her she was not a loser, but a success. She had one hiccup in her life, but that would not stop her from achieving greatness. She was out to prove to her family and her friends, she was better then her present circumstances and would do what ever it took to get ahead.

I do not remember the divorce of my parents. My earliest memory starts with the two of them separated. I only know what I have been told about the divorce and what transpired during those months when they had called it quits, going their separate ways. I found it to be very clear, my father tried to play the innocent man driven to an affair due to the constant nagging of his wife. He played off his role in the divorce as something caused because my mother did not understand him or was not encouraging and supportive like a wife should be.

My mother took on the role of a woman betrayed by the man she loved. Her love for him quickly became resentfulness, which in turn led to spite. She felt her family was looking at her in a mocking and unsupportive way, forcing her into a shell created by the embarrassment of her situation and the humiliation of her failures.

With the support of her friends at Nationwide, she turned her shame into a force which led her to freedom. No longer would she be dependant on what her husband was doing or what her family felt she should be doing. She was bitten by independence, her strength coming from the love for her two children. This was the beginning of her new life, completely separate from the old. With David still in diapers and myself still a toddler, she took her first step to the rest of her life. She flexed her newly found independent muscles with the divorce. She would show all of those involved who really had control over the situation and who was going to make her future and the future of her young children.

Divorces in the late seventies were not like they are today. They were not common place and were still considered a dirty secret people would not speak about. Divorce was a sign of shame, especially for the woman, but my mother did have the cards stacked in her favor. Her husband had been the cheating party giving her incredible grounds for the divorce. My father knew this—he was aware of what the courts could do if she so requested.

When my mother went into the divorce, she did not take everything. She could have, but she did not. Instead she requested all the assets the two of them had acquired be split between the two of them. She later explained to me, she did this primarily because she did not want anyone thinking she was living off her ex-husbands achievements. She took half of what they had, and that was good enough for her. No one would be able to say she was living the good life by the sweat of my father's brow. Both would leave the marriage with equal shares.

With the assets split, there were just a couple other issues to resolve. First, there was David and I. It was clear going in who would get custody of us, but it was unclear about visitation and child support. With full custody of David and me going to my mother, she requested support from our father. Being a studious mother she figured out what the cost of her two children would be on a monthly basis and split that figure in two. She asked for two-hundred and fifty dollars from my father per month to help with the responsibility of our care. Again she was very careful not to give my dad's supporters ammunition against her. She did not want anyone to come back to her and say she was inflating the child support so she could live in excess on my father's dime. She simply requested he pay half of the actual current cost of my brother and I. They had had us together, and she was willing to pay for the other half of the expenses.

Visitation to my father was given at my mother's discretion. She did not want a man who ran the roads, was lazy, and was filled with unfulfilled dreams around her children. She did not want his influence rubbing off on her two children. My mother never said no to my father when he wanted to see us, but she wanted the ability to do so if she felt it was needed.

When the judge gave full custody to my mother with visitation at her discretion, my father did not take it favorably. He saw this as a way for my mother to take his children away from him never to be seen again. He voiced his opinions by threatening death to anyone who tried to stop him from seeing us.

The judge asked my father what he would do if he told him he could not see his children, and my dad responded, with his attorney trying to cut him off, that he had a riffle and bullet with the judge's name on it. This was really the first time he showed his undying love for my brother and me. I do not think he saw what he had until someone decided to take it away from him. He may have hated my mother at the time, but he loved us. Unfortunately, the judge did not see in his comments the dedication he had to his two sons.

His attorney was able to play the Vietnam angle, and my dad was able to spend a few months in the Veteran's Hospital to undergo a psychiatric evaluation. He was lucky he was not held in contempt of court or even worse, forbidden to see his children by court order. I am sure my mother cracked a smile at the turn of events in the divorce proceedings. Until this point, my dad had looked at the divorce as a joke and completely my mother's fault. Finally, the severity of what was happening hit a cord with my dad.

David and I were never played to hurt our parents. My mother was not trying to use us as a tool to inflict emotional pain on my father. She was simply starting a new life and was completely severing the cord with the past. She did not want my father to have control of her fate or the fate of her children. Even with that said; I know she enjoyed seeing the pain on his face. The divorce was not enough to hurt him the way he had hurt her, but this had.

Assets had been divided; custody and visitation had been established. The only thing left was alimony. My mother had a clear plan for alimony. It is customary for this to be used to help the hurt party in a marriage to maintain a standard of living similar to that while in the marriage. I am positive my dad and those who supported him thought she was going to go deep with this portion of the divorce. My mother's friends and family thought this would be were she would get back at my dad for his adultery; but that is not how she was thinking.

My mom did not want my father's money. If she had she would have asked for more in child support or more of their mutual assets. She was entitled to more due to the circumstances of the divorce, but she simply wanted to completely sever ties with my father, but never let him forget what he had done. Custody and visitation was the first reminder to my father, and she used alimony as her second reminder to him.

My mom requested ten dollars a month in alimony payments from my father until she either was remarried or until her death. This meant my dad was going to be making an alimony payment of ten dollars to my mother for the rest of her life. It was not enough to do much more then buy a dinner at McDonald's, but it would be a reminder to him of their marriage, and the mistakes he had made towards her.

Taking such a small amount would again, protect her from those thinking she was taking advantage of the situation and digging into my father for the money he had at the time and the money he would potentially be earning in the future. When everything was over and the divorce final, no one could say my mother took anything more the ten bucks a month from my father. Everything else had been split up evenly between the two of them. From this point on, anything made in life was of her doing. My dad would not have anything to do with it.

With the divorce behind her, she purchased a small house off Alabama Avenue in Lynchburg. She purchased new furniture, and set up her new home along with her new life to her liking. Her life was just beginning, and she started with the intentions of providing everything needed to raise her children and to make it in the business world.

This new house would hold the very first memories I can recall. Though it is fragmented, as most memories from when a person was three years old, I know I was living in a loving household where all my needs were met.

9

The Beginnings of a New Life

Starting out on her own, my mother dove herself into her work. Nationwide Insurance and the people working with her became her new family. Those employees became her backbone in life, and her job was her way up in life. After the divorce, she not only gained her freedom, but gained full responsibility of two small children who were just starting to become active in life.

For the most part, David and I were just babies when my parents were married. Not really walking or getting into much trouble. There was one incident when I had awaken early one morning and went into the kitchen to get something to eat. David was still just hobbling around, just learning to walk. When I went into the kitchen that morning, I did not want cereal; I wanted bacon. Being the studious little man, I pulled up a chair to the stove, turned on the burner (This was before the controls to the burners were placed on the back of the stoves. The controls were right up front where I could reach them.), and dropped some bacon into the pan. I had seen Mom cook bacon many times, and I felt I was ready to do it myself.

To my surprise, the stove caught on fire from all the grease the pound of bacon was producing as it cooked all at once. With the flames lapping up the wall behind the stove, I went into my parent's bedroom and told them there was a problem with the stove. It was way too hot and burning my bacon.

Their heads cleared from the night's sleep instantly with the smell of smoke. It ended up that I burn half the kitchen before the fire was put out. I can not remember the incident, but I was told the story many times when I tried to cook or tried to do anything that dealt with something hot or a flame.

This happened on Newbern Street, but at our new home on Alabama Avenue, I had a new buddy to get into trouble with. David was finally old enough to do many of the things I could do. My mother could have never expected what two small boys could get into or what it would take to keep an eye on us. Prior to the divorce, David and I were fairly easy to control. Now a new chapter in her motherhood had begun. We were both able to talk, open doors and windows, and dig through drawers and cabinets.

Our new house had a backyard that butted up to a wooded valley. In that wooded valley were trails that led to a school on the other side of the ravine. This school had a playground and it became my mission to play in that playground.

Dad came over soon after mom bought the new house and put up a chain-link fence so we could play out back and would stay in the yard where mom could keep an eye on David and me. The fence was about four feet high with the only way in or out of the fenced area through the back door of the house. It served the purpose of keeping our dog Bow in (Noisy had died a few months earlier) and keeping stray animals out.

I saw this as a challenge. I did not want to play in the fenced in area. I wanted to play in the trees and bushes on the other side of the fence. It was my mission to get over that fence and into the freedom of the woods. It looked so much more fun than the kiddy pool and swing set I had to play on inside the fenced area.

One afternoon Mom had stepped into the house for a moment to answer the phone or the door, I can not remember which, and I seized the opportunity. With David in tow, I climbed over the fence and headed into the woods—Bow yapping as he watched us disappear into the brush.

It was no trouble at all finding the trails in the woods that wound their way through the trees and brush, and David and I started out to explore what the fence had tried to keep us from. The dirt hardened walkway eventually led out to the playground of the school on the other side. We had discovered a place where we could play on sliding boards, seesaws, swings, and be completely free from the watchful eye of our mother.

Whatever she was doing before she stepped out just moments after leaving, she immediately stopped when our mother noticed we were gone. Her stomach had to have leapt into her chest as she scanned the area to see if we had just moved to a play area out of her direct sight. She was unable to find us and the panic started to hit home. She called out our names, but we were too far and having too much to have heard her.

After her yells did not produce her two children, she quickly called my dad and he was over within just moments. While waiting, my mom went out front, walked up and down the street looking for her two wondering children, but turned up empty handed. She never thought to go into the woods behind the house.

When Dad showed up, he immediately went into the woods. He had always been the most playful parent and seemed to understand the lure of the woods beyond our backyard. He followed the trails and quickly came to the school yard David and I were happily playing in. I do not remember what he did or said when he saw us playing, while our mother was loosing her mind, but I imagine he had some choice words for us, and he quickly took us back home.

It was just a few days later, when the fence grew from about four feet to roughly ten feet. My dad had to make it too tall for David and me to climb. This did not really do any good. I figured if I could not climb the fence, I would just dig under it. It was just a few weeks after we had first climbed the fence, when David and I began digging under the fence to get out. We were determined to play in the playground just a short distance from out backyard. A fence, no matter how tall, would not stop us.

After the second escape, it became a rule that we could not play out back without someone directly watching us. If mom had to step back in the house, we had to follow. No longer could we play in the backyard, plotting our escapes from the fenced area to obtain freedom just beyond the woods.

Our lives had changed along with our mother's life. David and I were now starting to walk and talk and the world was a place to be explored and to be played in. No longer were we unable to open cabinets, or doors, or root around through draws. We had been freed with the ability to move upright, and we did just that. Escaping from the fenced in yard was just the beginning of the exploration David and I would do at our new house as we grew into out new lives.

Mom was working hard at Nationwide to provide the very best for us. She worked most of the day and not wanting us to be left with our dad for care during the day; she enrolled us in our first day care.

Called the Busy Bee on Fort Avenue in Lynchburg, I can still remember my time there. Mom would drive us there early in the morning, around seven or so, and leave us in the care of the staff. Before leaving though, she would come to the window of our class room and blow us a kiss as a reminder she would be back when work was over to take us home.

Being a logical and systematic mother, Mom had chosen Busy Bee because of it's location to her work. Nationwide was just up the street and close enough for her to get to her children in an emergency or to come over at lunch to have a peek at the treatment of her children.

With us at daycare she was able to put her complete efforts into her work and into our futures. She was working not only for herself but for the well being of David and me. The center of her life had changed from the relationship with my father and her former marriage, to the care and happiness of her two children. We had become the axis by which her world turned.

Life in our new home had fallen into a routine. David and I would go to day-care, and mom would go to work during the day. Or lives had structure and a purpose. Security was now starting to form around us, and the world seemed to be a little brighter.

David and I still got into everything around the house. I can remember getting a nice talking to about the toilet and how I was not allowed to flush it unless I used it. It would seem our water bill came due at over a hundred dollars, and I was unaware that every time I flushed the toilet we were being charged for the water used. I just liked to hear the rush of the water and watch it as it went down the drain.

Bedtime also became a problem in our new life. David and I rarely wanted to go to sleep when Mom said we had to. I shared a room with David at the time and Mom would tuck us into bed way before we thought it was time to go to sleep. If she got to stay up late, we did not see why we could not stay up late too.

Of course, as soon as she shut the door, David and I would get out of our beds and play with the toys in our room. On many occasions we were too loud and Mom heard, quickly putting a stop to our fun time after bedtime. Eventually she started leaving our bedroom door open so she could see if we turned on our bed-room light to play. She could also hear us more clearly as we hopped out of bed to play with out trucks or building blocks.

It became a battle between us and our mom. She wanted us to go to sleep, and we wanted to stay awake. Since playing in our room became too risky because we could get caught, we started sneaking out of our room and playing elsewhere. David and I would creep out of our room, past the den where Mom was working or watching TV into the living room where we could play without being heard. Like every house where there are little kids, toys were everywhere. Playing in the living room was no different then playing in our bedroom. We just had a slip by Mom and not turn on any lights. The creeping around actually made it more exciting.

We were caught on the first night we tried to sneak into the living room. We never figured she would go to the kitchen for something during the night. She had to walk through the living room to get to the kitchen, and she walked right into David and me playing with our cars and G.I. Joes. Back to bed we went.

The next night we did the same thing, but Mom checked in on us several times and when she saw we were gone, she came and got us and put us back in bed. Each time she had more and more choice words with us to let us know how annoyed she was. For a few days we stayed in our room when she put us to bed, but during those few days we made some plans. We plotted how we could get past her and not get caught. We decided to hide when we heard her coming, and then try to sneak back into the bedroom while she was looking for us.

The very next night we put our plan into action. When Mom saw we were not in our room, she came into the living room but did not see us. We hid pretty well behind the sofa, but left our toys in the middle of the floor. When she went into the kitchen, we slithered out and headed to our room, the sound of running feet on hardwood echoing throughout the house. Of course, she caught us halfway, long before we made it to our room.

This was the last time this was going to happen. She thought she had a way to fix the dilemma of her two rambunctious sons. When she put us back in our beds she tied the door shut with a jump rope. The jump roped allowed the door to be open just enough so she could peak in but we could not get out.

This seemed to work. Every night after that she would tie the door shut. Before she went to bed, well after we had fallen asleep, after many protests to be let out because we did not want to go to bed, she would take the rope off and open the door.

She thought she had the problem solved, but David and I took things to an even higher level. If we could not sneak out through the door, there were two windows to use. Being the oldest and the tallest since I was four, I took on the role of the hero that found a way out. David, being just two, was not tall enough to get up to the window so I would have to leave him behind.

After being tucked in for the night, David and I went into action. We waited a few minutes to make sure Mom was in the other room doing whatever it was she did while we were sleeping. When the coast was clear, we piled all the pillows on my bed, giving me just enough of a boost to reach the window and open it.

Very quietly, I unlocked the window and slid it open. The screen was a bit of a problem but eventually I got it out of the way and was ready to crawl through to the night outside. David helped by placing a large fire engine on the bed for me to get my final boost so I could get through the window. Both of us checked to make sure Mom was not paying attention, and then I went through. I climbed through the window and into the bush just outside, David left behind, just barely able to see over the window sill.

With just a little maneuvering, I was free from the bush and standing in our front yard in my pajamas. I was fortunate enough to be wearing the zip up pajamas with the feet in them. David and I had a conversation through the window for a few moments, before I decided it was time to get back inside.

Getting out was the plan, we never thought about how I would get back in. I tried the bush, but I was not able to climb it high enough to get back in. David tossed out the bed spreads thinking I could climb back in using it as a rope, but nothing worked. It was getting dark, and I could not get back in.

I went around back and squeezed through a space under the fence we had dug earlier and tried the back door. It was locked and with Bow barking like a crazy dog, I went back under the fence and to my bedroom window, where David was waiting. The bush was now filled with toys and the sheets and bed spreads from our beds.

Panic was starting to set in so I went to the front door and rang the doorbell. Mom quickly came to the door and found me standing on the porch looking up at her caked with dirt. She quickly picked me up and went to our bedroom to check on David. It did not take her long to realize what we had done. There was a pile of pillows and toys leading up to the window, and the bushes outside were filled with items used to try to get me back into the room without her knowing. This was the first yelling I can remember. We had crossed a line, and she definitely let us know it.

Some time went by before we tried an escape from bedtime again. When we did attempt it again, our dad was waiting for us outside. He had stopped over to drop of some things to our mother after work. It was roughly nine at night and as he was walking up to the front door to ring the bell when he noticed the movement of flashlights outside our bedroom window.

Knowing the flashlight beam was pointed at the room where his two children slept and being the protective dad, he immediately went over to investigate. What he found was me in the bushes and David half hanging out the window. We had used more things to get him up high enough so he could get out with me this time.

Dad quickly scooped up David before he tumbled to the ground and lifted me out of the tangles of the bush. We were always excited about seeing dad; we did not understand what had happened or why he was not living with us. He was always excited to see us as well and would do anything to see us smile. Dad also meant fun and we knew this. With the two of us in his arms, we asked him to take us to get some candy.

Not thinking what would happen when Mom checked on her two sons and they were not in their beds, dad took us to the 7-Eleven to get candy. We never told Mom we were leaving; we just piled into Dad's car and headed for the store.

We were only gone a few minutes. The store was just up at the top of the street, but it was getting late. Mom was tired and was getting ready to go to bed. She took the rope off our door and peeked in to discover we were not in the room, the window wide open.

She went outside to look for us, but it led to nothing. We were nowhere to be found. She awoke the neighbors calling for us and even went to the playground beyond the woods looking for us, but she never found us.

After frantically searching outside she turned to inside the house, but still came up empty handed. She was dialing the police when the three of us walked into the house. David had his bag of candy and I had mine. We even made sure we bought some for Mom, but she did not seem happy about the Raisonetts we brought her.

This was the first spanking I can remember. We had taken our escape tactic to a new level, and she took her punishment to a new level. She never hurt us, but with the fact she was upset and smacked us across the legs, tore David and me up. We were so sorry for what we had done. We also blamed everything on Dad. He was the one who took us to get candy.

I can not remember what she did or said to Dad but I know it was far worse then anything she ever said to us. That night before tucking us in for the second time, she nailed both windows shut. We would no longer be climbing out during the night via our bedroom window. With all our escape options depleted, David and I conceded to our mother's request for us to go to sleep when she told us to.

Even though she had problems getting us to stay in bed and going to sleep, all I ever had to do to get her to come to me at night was call her name. It was like she had super sonic hearing. Anytime I had a bad dream or was afraid of the dark I just had to call her. She would either come into my room and comfort me or pick me up and put me in her bed to sleep for the night.

Though she would gladly put us in her bed when we were scared, she learned very quickly to make sure we did not have anything in our mouths before laying us down. One Saturday morning she found the gum I was chewing before going to bed in her hair. After that she systematically took all gum and candy from our room so we would not get into it after bedtime. Dad always restocked us, but Mom was aware of the potential catastrophe after having to cut the gum from her hair, so she did what she could to keep it from happening again.

I can remember many nights I would crawl into her bed at night after having a bad dream or hearing something in the night that spooked me. No matter how mad we made her, or how much trouble we gave her, she always extended her love to us. She always made us feel safe.

As time passed, the memories of having two parents together started to fade, and David and I forgot what it was like to have Dad living with us. Though it faded from our minds, it was still in our mother's, and those memories were still painful and impossible to get away from in Lynchburg. Everywhere she went was a reminder of the failure she had in her marriage.

She was learning to be a mother and was doing well at her job, but she did not feel free from her mistakes and from those who were looking down on her. It was time to take the next step and to truly start a new life.

It was time for her to leave her home and start a new life. She had taken the first step into becoming her own person, and it had come time to take the next step. This one would be far harder and a lot more risky then leaving her husband.

10

Leaving the Old to Start Something New

It has been said time heals all wounds, but in my mother's case, time just seemed to add to the loss she experienced with her marriage. Everyone knew her past; she was unable to escape and start over living in Lynchburg, Virginia. She had to get out to move on.

Since her divorce, her younger sister, Wanda, had moved out west in pursuit of a better life with her husband and children, and her older sister, Doris, was doing well with her three children and husband. She saw herself as the inferior member of the family. She considered herself not to be good enough to be a part of her own family. Her two sisters were happily married, and she was left alone raising two boys.

She was not able to separate herself from my dad. Every time she turned around, he was there. He was always prying into her affairs and into the affairs of her two children. The woman who had been her neighbor and friend, who eventually became my father's extramarital lover, was always throwing the loss of her husband in her face. She could not free herself from the hurtful past.

Internally, she was screaming to get away—to leave her old life behind to start over afresh. She could not start over carrying the baggage of the past and decided to leave that baggage in Lynchburg, once and for all. Through her hard work at Nationwide, my mother was offered a job at the home office in Columbus, Ohio. This was her chance to get far away from the problems of the past and start over in a new place with new faces and new opportunities. I do not know how long it took her to make the decision, but I do not think it took long when she saw she had the potential to build a future for herself and her children.

It is unclear as to what the reaction to her leaving was like for her and her family. I was too little to remember, but I do remember a time with my dad after she had told him. He had come over to visit in one of his vehicles he hoped to restore and sell for a profit. When he got back in the car to leave, it would not start. The alternator had given out, and it would not turn over.

With a disgusted grunt he got out, popped the hood and began removing the faulting alternator. I can remember this day like it was yesterday. I was allowed to go outside with dad as long as I stayed out of the way and did not run off like I had the habit of doing. It gave Mom some time to catch her breath.

It was the first time it was just me and Dad doing guy things, just the two of us. He sat me up on the fender and talked to me while he cussed the alternator out of car. He asked me if I understood what it meant to be moving to Ohio and what I thought about it. I was just four so I did not have much to say, other than I would miss him and asked him to come and visit all the time.

He said he would as he continued to take out his frustrations on the faulting car part. Eventually, after snapping off the bolt in the process, the alternator was free and ready for the new one.

Just like at our house on Newbern, Dad had some spare parts in the basement to handle a problem just like this. It was just one of the many reminders of the man Mom once married. I do not understand why she let him keep some of his things at her house, but she did. He brought the replacement alternator from the basement placed it in the car to ensure it was actually a fit.

He still needed to run up to the auto part store to get some replace bolts and asked if I want to go. I declined, and he went on in my mother's car. While he was gone, I decided to help him out a bit with his problem. I could tell he was upset and wanted to make things better for him. I did not understand the words he was saying, but I knew they were words of frustration and sadness.

Sitting in the driveway with Dad's new alternator, I went to work. I would have it apart in no time for him. With a screw driver and a hammer, I banged and pried until I had his replacement part in about ten pieces, all ready for him when he got back.

Mom did not know I had been left alone in the driveway. Dad had not told her I had been left out there. She was under the assumption I was at the store with him. I did not have any idea I was not supposed to take the alternator apart with a hammer and screw driver. I am not even sure how I was able to it, but toddlers can surprise you sometimes. When Dad returned I was standing in the drive in my overalls, covered in grease, with a big grin across my face.

Dad saw what I had done before he had to ask, but he asked anyway. I told him I had helped him out while he was at the store. Everything was ready for him to fix his car. With out hesitation, he picked me up, hugged me and told me thank you. He told me I had really helped him out and that he was proud of me.

He never let on that I had destroyed his alternator and that a new would have to be bought to replace the one I had hammered into multiple pieces. He took me in the house and gave me to Mom—surely frowning from the looks of her greasy son, and told her he would be back in a little bit. He still needed some parts from the auto center.

This was the only time I can remember ever discussing Ohio with Mom or Dad. This is also one of my most memorial memories I have of my dad. He truly made me feel special that day. It also seemed to give him some assurance regarding the move, knowing I was not upset about leaving and was willing to do whatever I thought it was take to make him happy.

Even though he knew the move would be a good opportunity for his children, he did not want us to go—even argued against it. He was seeing those most important to him leaving, and he was one of the main reasons. He had screwed up, and the consequences of his actions were now starting to catch up in a way that tore deeply at his heart.

Mom visited Ohio for her interview and everything went over with flying colors. While she was gone during one of her visits to Ohio, our dad watched over us along with a teenage girl named Lori. Lori had babysat for us in the past, and she and her family would be a familiar face in Ohio, for they were moving also in pursuit of a better life.

David and I loved it when she watched over us while mom worked late or went out for the evening with her friends. She was a cool babysitter. I can remember her making cookies for us, but instead of making normal size cookies, she just took the entire roll of cookie dough and pressed it onto the cookie sheet—one giant cookie.

When they were done, she cut the enormous mass of chocolate chip into four sections. David and I could not have just one cookie; we had to have a cookie in each hand. The pieces were larger than our heads, and we thought we had found heaven. We were not able to eat even half of one of the pieces, but just holding them was more then enough for us to be overly thrilled. Mom was not too happy when we would not go to sleep from being on a sugar high, but she did not seem to mind. We liked Lori, and she treated us well. That was all Mom was concerned about. Lori became a regular with David and I, and that relationship continued into our future home in Ohio.

When Mom returned from Columbus, she came back with a job offer and a way out. For the next several weeks, we were getting ready to move. She was preparing to leave her entire life; to go to a place where she just knew the few who had also received new jobs. She did not know the area; she did not even have a place to live, but she had determination.

It was early spring when we left for our new home. The three of us piled into the car and headed northwest. Everything we knew, our father, our aunts and uncles, and our cousins, all left behind. From this point on David and I would grow up with a new set of friends and make such dear friends we would consider them our family over those we left in Lynchburg.

11

Strangers in a new Place

The drive through the mountains to the endless fields of corn and soy took what seemed like a lifetime. David and I fidgeted in the car waiting to get to our destination. This was before the West Virginia Turn Pike was in place, and the drive was mainly on two lane roads that twist and turned through the steep mountains. Traffic was backed up in many places as we waited to make it through one lane roads surrounded by the construction of the new freeway to come.

After ten hours in a car, we finally made it to Columbus. It was bigger than anything David or I had ever seen. The tall buildings of downtown wowed us we looked up at the lights shining through the windows several hundred feet above us. The size of the city was daunting to us. Lynchburg was simply a very small town in comparison. Though it was by far the biggest city in the country, David and I were certain that Columbus was the biggest.

The fascination of the city took a back seat to our tiredness from the long drive, and Mom quickly settled us into a hotel room for the night. Our first night in Columbus was spent at the Red Rooster Inn just off RT-161 not far from the Continent and French Market. At the time, this was the very center of everything in Columbus. It was the place to be, and the place to be seen.

Mom did not have much time to get everything settled before her work started at her new job. With this time crunch to worry about, the next day she arranged to enroll David and I at a daycare center just down the road called The Little Buckeye. This would be the place where we would spend our time from six in the morning to about six at night while she worked hard to start our new lives.

Since she had left in such a hurry—the job mandated she began soon—she did not have much money. She barely made it to Columbus and paid for the hotel room. Without any money in here pocket, she was unable to get us an apartment right away. We were all going to be stuck in the small hotel room for a couple of weeks until she received her first couple paychecks.

I do not know how she made things work these first few weeks. When I look back and I think about having to pay for the hotel room, the childcare, the food, and other expenses, I can not figure out how she made her finances work. I am sure a great deal of it went on credit, but I know it was tough for her.

In addition to these stresses, it did not take David and I long to figure out we were not going to see anyone we knew for quite some time. Until this point, everything had been an adventure, but soon we were ready to go home. We wanted to see those we loved and were familiar with. We did not want to be around these strangers all the time.

We did not understand—we were looking at the world and the events around us through the eyes of children, and it started to scare us. This was too much for the two of us, and we started to let her know this. David and I both acted out and whined and cried. We did whatever we could to make it clear we did not like what she was doing. We wanted to go have dinner with Dad and play with our toys.

We did not have any toys in this hotel room, and we had become tired of eating lunch meat from Big Bear and cookies from the vending machines. We were ready to go home. In fact, insisted on going home. I can remember some very specific moments in that hotel room and do not know how my mother did what she did. Though David and I were acting out in every way we could think of, including not going to sleep, crying out for our dad, not eating anything she bought for us, she never yelled at us. She simply told us, everything would be ok. We would have our toys soon, and Dad would be visiting as soon as we had a place.

She had an understanding; we were just children and did not know what was happening or really why we had left home. She was extremely careful not to let the stresses of her life come out in the way she handled David and I. We were completely unaware she was broke; she was scared, and was second guessing herself. In a hotel room this was very hard to do. There was no place for her to go without seeing the two of us.

The few times she talked about our time in the hotel when we first moved here, she told me that was the time in which she made a vow to succeed. Though we were not exactly the most lovable children at the time, just being around her so much constantly pounded into her the reason she had made such a radical change.

When she first left Lynchburg, her motives had been to start over with her life and to build something that was hers and hers alone. Living in that hotel room for a month and seeing that her actions directly affected her two children, forced her motives into a completely new direction. David and I became the sole purpose of her life. To make us smile was all she ever worked for. Instead of working her way out of the failures she had experienced in her marriage and working for a better life for her children, my mom completely submitted herself to the love and success of her two boys.

After a couple of weeks we settled into a routine that became the norm while we were staying in the cramped hotel. David and I spent our days at The Little Buckeye, and Mom worked hard at her new job. Though a routine had been established, day to day life was rough. The home sickness was setting in for all three of us. The newness of Mom's new job started to fade, and the reality of what she had done sank in deeper and deeper.

During this time our nights were spent solely at the hotel with the infrequent breaks of going to the grocery store to pick up food for the next few days. This pattern lasted for several weeks and was finally broken by the first few paychecks from Nationwide. These first few paychecks started to make it clear the move would work. There were still many tough times ahead, but the result would be worth the hard work. The cloud of doubt that was beginning to fill my mother's mind, started to fade slightly.

Her money came exactly at the right moment, and it was more than enough to get us out of the hotel room and into a townhouse. It was also enough to move our stuff from Lynchburg to our new home in Columbus. Some of the things we were familiar with were coming to us to provide some comfort in a time of server insecurity.

I remember very well this move. It was the first part of April and it was snowing while we set everything up in our new place. It did not snow much in Lynchburg, and it definitely did not snow during this time of the year. It did not last very long and melted just a few days after falling, but it gave David and I a chance to play outside with other kids from the complex—something we had not done for a while.

With the joys of the snow, also came the fascination of the new apartment. Though it was only a two bedroom, it was enormous to David and I. We had a huge basement, and we were able to have our own beds, instead of sharing a bed like in the hotel room. The apartment looked different on the outside, compared with our house in Lynchburg, but on the inside it was the same. All our toys were now strung throughout the house, the furniture was all there and in its place, and we were able to have hot food to eat. Macaroni and Cheese with hotdogs never tasted as good as they did at this new place of ours.

A new invigoration entered our lives. We were now someplace we could call our own. We had room to play and all the toys we needed. Life had been looking grim, but it was turning around. Things were starting to look a little better. Home sickness still loomed in our hearts, but new friends were being made, and Lynchburg was beginning its fade to the past.

To help relieve the desire for home, Dad came for a visit. It was his first visit to Ohio, and I know David and I were thrilled to see him. Though, she would not admit it, I know my mom was just as happy to see someone from home. David and I were young and able to let go of Lynchburg far easier then she would be able to. She had too many memories to simply forget, and seeing my dad brought a piece of her past back to her in a time when she needed to be reminded and comforted in respects to her bold life changing decisions.

As the summer approached, Dad spent more and more time in Ohio with us. He did this to help out with cost of childcare. Mom was saving to purchase a home and a permanent place for her children to grow up. She wanted to do this before I started Kindergarten and that was just a year away. It was also nice to have another adult around to talk to, as opposed to a four and three year old.

This summer with Dad was a great summer filled with exploring the new city. I can remember going and seeing The Dark Crystal and Bambi with him. The Dark Crystal scaring me and giving me nightmares, and Bambi making me cry when Bambi's mom died. We spent a lot of time at the malls and were fascinated as to how big they were. We also just spent time driving around the city and looking at the new places.

We found the lake at Alum Creek and spent many days playing in the sand and swimming off its beaches. Mom was spending more time with her new found friends at her job, and we were introduced to a whole new group of people. For David and I, home had moved to Ohio, but Mom still considered home back in Lynchburg and was struggling with settling into her new life.

Our first Christmas rolled around along with the magic that came with the holidays. Everything seemed to be new and a complete mystery that needed to be explored. The city of Columbus was a fairy tale city for David and I, filled with all the wonders of Christmas magic. The anticipation of the visit from Santa was enough to keep us up late at night on a constant excitement rush.

When asked what we wanted for Christmas, David and I unanimously agreed on a gorilla. Earlier in the fall we had been taken to the Columbus Zoo—saw more animals that we had ever seen before. There were baby gorillas playing in their environment, and we both wanted one as a pet. They seemed like a fun thing to have as a new addition to our home. Every time we sat on Santa's knee we asked adamantly for the gorilla.

Through the month of December, Mom made efforts to get us to look at some toys, or to look at some other items besides the gorilla, but we did not want anything else. It took a lot of convincing on her part to get us off the gorilla gift. If I remember right, she told us Santa had looked, but all the gorillas he had wanted to go back to their parents. She told us that Santa had to let his gorillas go home so they would be happy. It was a thin excuse, but it worked for David and I. We did not want the gorillas to be away from their family, and we could visit them at the zoo anytime we liked.

We ended up getting toys we loved and played with and completely forgot the loss of the gorilla. We totally forgot when we came down early that Christmas morning and saw fire trucks, stuffed animals, Star Wars action figures all heaped under our Christmas tree.

With the pass of our first holiday season, we had grown accustomed to living in Ohio. David and I had forgotten most of our past and the people in our past. With the exception of Dad, many of our family members, if not totally forgotten, became a distant memory of people we once knew. Mom was still clinging to the past, but it was starting to fade from her memory as well. Her friends at Nation-wide filled the gaps in regards to her relationships left in Lynchburg. She was in the process of making new friends and extended family and her efforts were starting to show results. She no longer felt completely alone. She now had others to lift the weight of loneliness.

There were problems throughout our first year in Columbus, but we had made it. Now my mother was looking towards the long-term future. Making good money, and being able to sell her home in Lynchburg, she was now able to pursue the task of obtaining a house we would build into a home.

Major hurtles had been over come, but she wanted to be someplace long-term before I started school. She needed to purchase a house soon. I was starting school next fall. This was a problem she took on head first and conquered her home buying dilemma—the final step to cutting off her past and starting a new life.

12

My Home Was Purchased

When our change to Ohio first took place, the goal was simply to start working and start bringing in money, living in a hotel until other arrangements could be made. When that was completed, and moving in a forward direction, it was time to get out of the hotel and into a more suitable living situation.

Now that Mom had rented a place to stay and had stabilized the daily routines of life, it was getting time to make a permanent move and solidify her commitment to David and I and to her new career. Purchasing a house was not only a more desirable living situation for us, but it was also a symbol of integration into our new lives. Purchasing a house meant selling our home in Lynchburg. It meant committing to a new home, making it hard to go back to Lynchburg. It would almost be impossible to go back once this was done. This was a life long decision not to be entered into lightly or without careful planning.

Mom wanted to get into a home before I started school. She did not want to be moving around while either David or I were in school. She understood the need to make new friends and not leave those friends simply because we no longer lived in the school area. We had already had to leave everyone we knew. While her friends remained relatively the same because she always went to the same place for work, David and I would be making friends at school. Moving us often would require the need to remake friends each time we moved. She did not want us to have to do this. One move during childhood was enough.

She also wanted someplace where David and I would stay out of trouble. We had already shown we were going to get into things and not do what she told us to do on a regular basis. Lynchburg was a relatively small city, so if we snuck out to play in the play ground the threat was relatively low, but Columbus was a different city and much larger. She also wanted a place where it would be easy to meet others. The big city sometimes hindered this. Starting out at a new job, cost was also a factor. She sought something she could afford and have plenty of room for all of us to stretch out without getting in the neighbors way or having the neighbors getting in our way.

With these things in mind, she began the daunting task of finding a place that met all of her needs but also allowed for growth as David and I grew. She started this just after the New Year and continued until she found what she was looking for. She was careful not to take David and I with her when she went out looking. She did not want us falling in love with a house she knew was not right. This could possibly lead her to purchase something that David and I liked and not something that would have everything we needed. She did not want to cave to our desires. Since her motives for working and for starting her new life now had David and I at the very center of her decision making, this could have been a real possibility if we went with her.

She did involve Dad with the decision on the new home. They had purchased several homes together when they were married, and he had a good eye for problems, and his advice to her always seemed to have the well being of his two children in mind. He was biased towards his two boys and looked at every house as the place where his two sons would grow up.

Between the two of them, it just took a couple of months for them to find a place that was affordable, had plenty of space, and fit into the lifestyle they wanted to provide to their two young children. They put the house into a contract, and with a little negotiating, closed on the deal just before the Easter holiday.

Satisfied his ex-wife had purchased a new house that was suitable for his sons, Dad went back to Lynchburg with peace of mind and an assurance we were never going to come back. Mom did not immediately tell David and I she had purchased a new house, instead she arranged it to be a surprise. This was the first time in a while she had been able to give us a surprise and would be able to see our eyes light up as we found out.

We were oblivious to anything she was doing. Easter was just a few days away, and we were waiting in anticipation for the Easter Bunny and his basket of candy he would leave to us. We had participated in an Easter egg hunt at the Little Buckeye that Friday so expectations for the visit from the bunny on Sunday morning were fresh in our minds.

Mom asked David and I if we wanted to go out to breakfast after opening our Easter Baskets Sunday morning. She told us we would be able to have some of the candy after we had eaten. We agreed and went to bed Saturday night with the anticipation of waking to plastic baskets loaded with chocolate left in our living room from the magical bunny.

Early Sunday morning, we awoke and rushed downstairs to see what the bunny had left for us. The sun was just beginning to peak over the horizon as we tore down the stairs and frantically rushed into the living room. We stopped just as we made to the bottom of the stairs. Looking intently into the living room we saw nothing.

There was nothing in the living room. It took a moment for us to compose ourselves and move into the small dining room and kitchen—again coming up empty handed. The excitement in our faces was quickly converted to panic. Had we been forgotten? Had the Easter Bunny hidden our basket much like he did his eggs during the hunt? We did not know, but we were determined to find out.

Hearing us rummaging around, Mom came down the steps to see what all the commotion was about—her hair still tangled from sleep and her face still waking up to the early morning. We explained to her we were looking for the presents from the Easter Bunny, but had come up empty handed—disappointment now setting in.

She told us it was still early and maybe the Easter Bunny got a little behind. Maybe if we went upstairs and got ready to go out to eat, everything would alright. He would slip in while we were getting dressed. It had promise, but David and I now had the urges of doubt. We had been forgotten.

The three of us went back upstairs and got ready to go out—the silence of disappointment hung thick in our room as we quietly got dressed. When we had finished we went downstairs to check things out one last time before we left. Nothing—we had been left empty handed. It was now obvious we had been skipped. We had been forgotten by the bunny, our hopes crushed and our spirit broken.

We left that morning completely hopeless of ever finding anything left from the bunny. David and I got in the car, and the three of us went out to breakfast. Mom tried to bring up our spirits, but nothing changed the fact we had not received our baskets filled with candy. After breakfast, Mom suggested we go for a ride in the country. Dad and her were looking at a new house, and she wanted us to have a look at it. It was still a possibility the bunny was running late. This would give him plenty of time to stop by our place while we were out looking at this new house.

At this point, David and I did not much care. We had just picked around our breakfast with the fear of receiving nothing for Easter becoming more and more a reality. Leaving McDonalds—the restaurant of choice for David and I—we began the half hour drive to the small town of Centerburg. We had never been there before and did not really want to go. We would have been more content going home and waiting, just in case our baskets were dropped by at a later time.

The drive seemed to take forever, and there was nothing to look at to break the boredom. Nothing but soy fields and corn fields for as far as the eye could see. Unlike Lynchburg, at the foot of the Blue Ridge Mountains, the country side of Ohio turned out to be a flat plate filled with the occasional house, but primarily dominated by fields freshly plowed by the farmer. To David and I there was nothing to look at out the window. Nothing to give us even the slightest glimmer of hope concerning why we had been left out by the bunny or to make this long drive a little more bearable to two broken hearted boys.

Finally, after riding in the car for a half hour, we came to the town of Centerburg. Mom seemed to be excited as we drove through town and told us about the house her and Dad were looking at. She never told she had already bought the house, but was hyping it up for when she did eventually tell us. I really did not care much about the new house. I just wanted to get there so I could get out of the car. I was tired of being cramped up with nothing to do but watch the unchanging scenery outside the window or playing with the few toys we had in the car.

It was apparent we were not going to be looking at a house within the Centerburg city limits. After passing through the few traffic lights Centerburg had, we headed out into the countryside again, but just for a few miles. Amidst several fields and between two houses sat a small home Mom had deemed suitable for us to grow up in. We pulled into the driveway and quickly got out of the car. The cramped car was making everyone a little agitated.

Mom asked us what we thought, and we shrugged our shoulders in indifference. We were too bummed out to care much. Seeing our sad faces, she walked up the small side walk, and we waited on the stoop as she unlocked the door and swung it open. She motioned for us to enter first, and we did with our heads hung low.

David was the first too spot them. Even though the house was empty of any furniture, I was looking at the floor, really not too interested in the house. With his shriek of elation I looked as well. In the middle of the bare living room were two of the largest Easter baskets I had ever seen.

They were both taller then the two of us and were loaded with candy and stuffed animals. Each one had a name on them. One said David, the other Christopher. We were really too shocked to go over to them. For the last hour or so we had pouted about not getting anything, and now it looked like we were left baskets bigger then we could had even imagined, even though it was in the wrong house.

We looked to Mom for reassurance as to what we were seeing. She explained to us that she must have made a mistake. Her and Dad had told the Easter Bunny to deliver the baskets here instead of to the apartment in Columbus. They thought we would be living here before Easter. She explained she was very sorry, but David and I had were not paying attention anymore. We were tearing at the plastic and tape trying to get at the candy and toys.

After a little help from Mom, we were into the baskets. Candy and stuffed toys now littered the floor of the empty living room. When we had quickly scarfed down a couple small items, it was now time to check out our new home. Our minds now in perfect harmony with the magic of the moment—the world now looked much brighter, and the home we had come to see now looked a lot more promising.

David and I were shown our new bedrooms. We would each have our own, something we had not had until this house, and we explored the rest of the house she had purchased to raise her children. This was a much better place then where we were living, and like our mom, could not wait to move in. The yard was huge as well—plenty of space for us to play with our trucks and toys. The whole place was filled with lots of opportunity for us to have lots of fun.

Within just a few days, our stuff was moved from Columbus to the small town of Centerburg. This would be the place where I would spend the majority of my childhood and grow up with those I met at school. This would become my hometown. The world was looking much brighter for all three of us. Moving into this new house was truly the beginning of a new life. There was no longer a turning back point for my mom, and it was the catalyst that made David and I products of Ohio and not of Virginia.

This house symbolized my mom's independence from those back in Lynchburg and a triumph over her failures. She was now planning her destiny, and things were falling in place. She was now in control of everything she did and was completely responsible for her own successes and failures. For David and I, Lynchburg was becoming even more distant. For her, the cord was slowly breaking, eventually to be left to memory.

The world was fresh to my family. The three of us were standing at the threshold to the foundation for the rest of our lives. None of us knew what lay ahead, but we all knew what we had left behind. The potential for our new future was greater than the destined future surely expected had we stayed in Lynchburg.

Every day that now past was a day in which our roots dug deeper into our new lives in Ohio.

Centerburg would be the place I would grow up; the place I would think of as home throughout the rest of my life. No matter where I went after this point, I would always look back to small town of Centerburg as my home and where I came from. I may not have been born there, but my spirit was firmly planted.

PART II
Raising the Average American Son

13

Centerburg Becomes Home

Located in the very center of Ohio, Centerburg was a small town when we first moved there in 1981 and is pretty much the same today. There are some new homes and a few new businesses, but in general, everything pretty much has stayed the same. With only three stop lights, one could drive through town without really seeing much. This is part of the town's magic.

The closeness of its people is the lure to those on the outside. It is a great thing to go to the gas station and see your neighbors and friends almost every time you fill up the tank. In the big city you are lucky to see anyone you know when you go out. The big city is simply too big to have that personal connection with its residences.

This small town setting was exactly what my mother was looking for when she set out to build a home for her two children. She wanted a homier place, as apposed to the conveniences of the suburbia. She also wanted a place to stretch out and have some privacy.

Our house in Centerburg was built on an old cornfield; the corn rows still lined the front and back yards. Behind our house was a cornfield, and we had neighbors on both sides far enough away for privacy but close enough for help if it was needed. Across the road from our house was a field cows used to graze during the long summer days.

This was the first time David and I had seen cows up close and on a regular basis. We had only seen cows a couple of times at a state fair or something of the like. So to have cows across the street was a great novelty for us. The neighbors just down the road had chickens, which at first was a curiosity but soon became somewhat of a nuisance. We did not know that roosters really do crow early in the morning. It did not matter if you were able to sleep in late; the rooster would still crow. It took at little while to get used to, but eventually we did and slept right through.

The house itself was exactly what one would suspect it would be like. It was a ranch style with three bedrooms, living room, dining room, kitchen, one and a half baths, and a two car garage. The yard was roughly four acres but very bare, formally being a corn field.

In comparison to what we had in Lynchburg, this place was a palace. Mom did not have to worry about us running off while playing outside. It would have been too far for us to really go anywhere. Since there were only cornfields around and no playgrounds, we did not have any reason to leave the yard. Plus, there were plenty of places to build forts, play with our toys, and lots of room to run around.

Dad came up for a few weeks to help Mom get moved in and to get the yard in decent shape. While mom painted the inside of the house, she sent Dad out to mow the grass. I am not sure what she was thinking when she sent him out to do the yard work. I guess she was just used to the small yards of her past, but this was several acres on ditch filled land, and all she had was a push mower. It took Dad a better part of a week to mow the grass that first time. With it being waste high, it had to be gone over several times to get it even close to being something presentable.

We all quickly learned about snakes and bugs. The country was filled with them. Every where we seemed to turn was a snake in the grass, or big grass hoppers jumping out of the weeds, and even worse—ticks. In Lynchburg, gnats and mosquitoes were the primary problem. Flies were common everywhere, but ticks were something new all together.

That first day of playing in the tall grass while Dad struggled to mow it, led to a night filled with Mom picking the ticks out of our dirty hair before we had our baths. After the frustrating task of having to wrestle two boys while she picked the blood sucking bugs off them, Mom made it clear we were not to play in the tall grass, and she wanted to look through out hair before we came in the house after playing. David and I did not disagree with her. We did not like having to have someone pick bugs off us anymore then she liked doing it.

In just a few days, we put everything into its place, and trimmed the yard into order. It still would take a good day or two to mow the entire yard with a push mower, but at least it would be easier to handle. All of our furniture was now in its place. David and I had set up our bedrooms, and our toys, and every other possession we loved, were around us. We settled into our new home very well. Other than the accents David and I still carried from the south, our home was in Centerburg. Lynchburg was simply a place we once lived.

While we were moving in, we had a few visitors from our past. Our former babysitter from Lynchburg had also moved to Centerburg. Lori, her sister Kristy, and their parents Don and Angie, bought a house just a couple miles down the road. Don and Angie both worked at Nationwide and had moved roughly the same time Mom had moved us. This family became her extended family that still had connections to her old life. They were her homesick comforters. Whenever she had problems, they were there to help her out. Or course, Lori was also there to help baby sit for David and I.

That first summer in Centerburg was spent almost entirely with Lori. She watched over us while Mom worked during the day. It was through Lori that I was able to see my school for the first time. She would be attending high school in the fall, and I would be starting Kindergarten. On many occasions she would have to go to the high school for various reasons, and she would take David and I with her.

I can remember the high school looking so huge and frightening. Even though the elementary school was smaller, it still looked huge to me, but a little friendlier. The high school was an old brick building like something out of a Boris Karloff film. The inside was even worse. The halls echoed as you walked, the ceilings were high and lined with pipes leading throughout the building, and there were no toys, or anything fun to do, just rooms lines with desks facing blackboards.

When she took me over to the elementary to look around, I felt better about going to school. There was a play ground. The building was only one level and seemed to be brighter, happier in its tone. Even through the high school loomed just a few hundred feet from the elementary, I took great solace in knowing I would be going to school in the cheerful school instead of the dark, huge halled building across the way.

School was still a few months away, and I was glad for it. I was not sure how I would like going to school in this new town. My friends were at The Little Buckeye. I would be starting over here. Everything would be new again. I could still remember the feelings I had when I started pre-school in Columbus, but at least there, David was a familiar face, someone I knew and could talk to if things with the other kids did not work out. Here I would be going by myself. I would be in a room full of strangers.

I had started out with a couple of fights at The Little Buckeye because of my accent. I was afraid the people in Centerburg would also make fun of the way I talked. If they did, I would not have David to talk to until I made friends; I would be alone. Though the building looked friendly, I was afraid of the people that would be in my class. My southern drawl was an easy target for anyone who wanted to poke fun. It was also giving me trouble learning to read. Mom had already taught me the alphabet and how to count, but the people in Ohio pronounced things differently. I had already dealt with this during my first few weeks at pre-school; I was not looking forward to it in Kindergarten.

Since Dad was here, I would have another great summer hanging out with him, and when he was not able to be here, Lori was there to take his place. They kept me busy that first summer. They took my mind off the fears of starting school in the fall. Lori was also as nervous as I was about starting school. She would be going to the gloomy high school in the fall with all kinds of new people. Her accent was just as bad as mine. I know she was thinking many of the same things I was.

Together, with David and her sister Kristy, we were able to drop our fears for a while and have fun in our new homes. Each of us made the others forget about the fears of the coming fall. The summer was a time of exploration and settling in for the long haul. All of us were here to stay, and it was time to start mingling with the locals; it was time to get out and see what Centerburg and the surrounding area had to offer.

That first summer is very vague to me; I can only really remember some trips to the park and to Mohegan to play in the river catching crawdads or simply floating with the currents. I do very clearly remember the lead up to my first day at school. It is interesting how I remember few of the new places I saw that first summer, but yet I clearly remember the week before school and the first week of school. After that first week, memories come and go until I enter the first grade.

14

The First Day of School

Dad came back to visit the week before my first day of Kindergarten. Lori was now busy getting herself ready for school and not able to watch David and I the entire time Mom was at work during the day. He would become our temporary babysitter until Mom made other arrangements.

Before actually starting school, Dad took me in for an orientation. I was able to see the class room where I would be learning and the teacher who would be teaching my class. I remember Mrs. Buxton very clearly to this day. She had such a sweet welcoming face and demeanor about herself. She was like the grandma everyone went to see on Sunday afternoons following church. I do not know how old she was, but to me she looked like a sweet old lady who would be sharing a part of herself to her class as the year progressed.

The classroom was just as you walked into the elementary school, just past the office across from the gym. I liked it being so close to the door. I did not want to have to walk any deeper into the school filled with strangers than I had to. I took comfort in the fact my escape would be relatively easy if the need should arise.

Dad, with David in tow, took me through me the room I would spend a half day each school day during the up and coming school term. I was thrilled to see the toys they had. It looked like a toy store with a play ground built into it. Everything was so bright and very cheerful. It did not look nearly as bad as what I thought it would.

While Dad talked with Mrs. Buxton, David and I were free to move around and explore the classroom. We also were able to meet some of the other kids who would be in the class with me. We were able to play with the others without the fear of being alone. Dad was just across the room. This gave me time to see if the others were going to share or if they were going to make fun of the way I talked. To my relief they did share, and they did not seem to notice I talked with a southern twang. We were equals as we played with our trucks on the carpeted roadways. That day of orientation relieved some of my fears of the new school.

When Dad was finished getting the list of supplies I would need and making sure all my paperwork was complete, we left for the day. I told my new friends goodbye and followed my dad back to the car. As I left that day, I did not realize some of the kids I met would be in my life for the next fifteen years and some even beyond that. These would be the people that would watch me grow up. I would be watching them grow up. Relationships would form, and then fall apart, only to be re-established much later. This group would become my extended family; they would help me with the problems life threw my way, and I would be there to help them. Some would become very dear friends; while others would simply become acquaintances remembered simply as someone I went to school with.

This kindergarten class would become the first chapter in my life and would introduce me to the people who would steer my life in many different directions as we together went from children to adult right before our own eyes. Though I had a past of only five years, these years spent in school would be the creation of my future and the way I fit into society as a whole.

Instead of going right home after leaving the open house at school, Dad took us out to get my supplies and to get lunch. He bought all the cool things I would need to make it through my first year. We bought crayons, watercolors, pencils, paper, a really cool Star Wars lunch box and matching back pack, and many other items I could not wait to use. With new friends, new supplies, and later new cloths when Mom came home, the excitement was starting to build. I could not wait for the big day when everything would come together. I would have a lunch packed, in my new cloths, and ready to use the crayons and watercolors Dad had bought. I could not wait. The fear of the unknown had somehow been replaced by the excitement of something new. I was looking forward to a day at school.

When the big day came, I was the first one up that morning. I could not wait to get to school. I dressed and ate as fast as I could. Of course, Mom redressed me when I spilt half my breakfast down my shirt from eating so fast. She also made sure I had my lunch packed and in my back pack ready to go. I do not know why I needed a lunch, considering I was only there for half a day, but it came in handy during snack time. It was only six thirty in the morning, and I was ready to go. Dad finally got up when I went into the living room and turned the television to cartoons and was bouncing around the room in excitement.

When the moment finally came, Dad took me to school. He walked me to the classroom and made sure my teacher saw that I was there. When he was satisfied everything was as it should be, he turned to leave. When he let go of my little hand and turned to leave, doubt rushed in. I was going to be alone with these new people. During orientation, everything had been different. Dad was just a shout away. Now he was heading out of the large glass doors, and I was being led into a room filled with those I did not know.

During that first day of class, Mrs. Buxton did most of the talking. She gave a detailed tour of the room and introduced each of us to the others in the class. That first day started very quiet and ended much more somber as all of us dealt with the same fears I was having. All of us were watching what the teacher was doing with nervous fears, wishing we could just go home.

That afternoon when class let out, the room cleared with a quick swift of students fleeing for the familiarity of their parents and anxious for the day to end, but as the days went on, everyone began to loosen up. We began remembering each others names; we began to play as if we had known each other all of our five years of life. Class now started with the roar of laughter and had to be settled each morning in order to hear the morning announcements and to say The Pledge of Allegiance we had just learned.

No longer did students run out to greet their parents at the end of the day. Many of us, including myself, had to be drug out in order to get us to leave. We all were friends and were having far more fun playing with fire trucks and blocks on the floor then going home to Mom and Dad. The fear of starting a new school, in a new town, quickly began to fade. I started to feel at home in this little town at the very center of Ohio.

After the first few days of school had passed, Mom felt confident enough to allow me to get on the bus in the morning instead of Dad taking me in every morning. He would still pick me up, but at least he did not have to drag David out of the house, and he had a little extra time to get things done before the bus came and picked me up. The bus now stopped at my house, and I got on every morning and headed to school.

As time passed, the help my dad was lending in getting me ready for school and caring for David and I while Mom was at work, was starting to wear thin. Mom was glad to have the little extra help, but she had moved to Ohio to get away from the man who now lived in her living room. The same problems that had crept into their marriage, now started to creep into her new life. They began to fight and to argue. They were never meant to be under the same roof. She had moved on to get away from that conflict, and now it was back.

Since Lori was not available, due to school, Mom was forced to look elsewhere for childcare. She had to work something out. Her ex-husband was unraveling the new life she had just started to build. As much as she had tried to prevent it, a piece of Lynchburg was rooted in the living room of her home in Centerburg. It had to be removed, and Mom set out to do this by arranging other forms of childcare for her two sons.

This search for alternative childcare other than my father led to one of the most unexpected surprises. Her quest for daycare led to the introduction of a woman who David and I would see as a grandmother, and Mom would see as an angel sent to ensure her new life was a success. This charming lady and her family replaced those we had lost by moving to Ohio. They replaced the aunts and uncles, cousins and grandparents of Lynchburg. They became the family my brother and I would grow up in, and the support our mother needed.

I do not know how Mom was introduced or how she discovered Marilyn, but as I look back on my life, some of my fondest childhood memories revolve around her and the time we spent with her and her family.

15

Mom Found an Angel

Marilyn opened the doors of her home to my family and really started the amalgamation into the Centerburg community. She was a pivot point in our lives that tilted the scales in favor of us and gave my mom the ability to do what she needed to build the future she wanted for her children.

Marilyn lived just across the street from the school in a large house that filled the Norman Rockwell imagery of small town life. The home was very welcoming and had the aurora of a time long past. You just knew Aunt Bee was in the kitchen cooking a hearty dinner. It was that kind of a place—almost magical in its sense of warm feelings.

Dad went back home to Lynchburg soon after Mom made other arrangements for the care of her two sons. He would be back to visit, but only on the occasion and not for any extended period of time. Marilyn now took the place of Dad and filled it with the likes of a loving grandmother who opened her life and heart to two small children from the south just as if we had been one of her own. She also gave her shoulder to our mother and offered her a friendly ear when Mom needed to talk.

With Dad gone, Mom had to get David and I ready and out the door in time for her to commute to Columbus without being late for work. She would get up around four-thirty in the morning, take her shower, do her hair, and put on her makeup. She always made sure David and I took our baths the night before so she would not have to worry about it that early in the morning. When she had finished her morning preparations for work, she woke my brother and I up and got us dressed—often times having to fight with us to get us out of bed at five-thirty in the morning.

After getting us to crawl out of our beds, getting us dressed was often far easier then combing our hair. I never could figure out what it was with the two of us, but we always seemed to wake up with hair filled with knots that took rigorous combing to get it into some kind of order. After getting us dressed, hair combed, she would put us in the car and drive us to Marilyn's in the dark mornings and drop us off. She would wait out front to make sure we made it up the steps and into the front door before pulling off to head south for work.

Each morning we would walk into Marilyn's to find her in her bathrobe making breakfast for her husband and her husband sitting at the kitchen table in his underwear sipping his early morning coffee. Both still looking haggard from a long nights sleep and being awakened rudely by an alarm clock. They both would greet us with a good morning, and we would head upstairs to catch a few more minutes of sleep before we had to go to school.

David and I would crawl into a warm bed and usually fall fast asleep only to be awaken an hour or so later by the Marilyn's yells at the foot of the steps for us to get up and come down for breakfast. By the time we made it to the kitchen the other children she was babysitting would already be digging into their bowls of cereal.

These other kids soon became friends to David and I. Most were our age, but a few were a little older. This table became a center piece of our friendships with one another. All of us sat there to eat, and this broke down all the barriers between us. We may be going to different classes at school, all came from different backgrounds, but at this table we were all the same. We were just a bunch of kids playing with our Rice Crispies and waiting for Marilyn to leave the room so we could really start the day off. When she was gone we had the opportunity to throw food, or play with toys on the table. With her standing over us, we were expected to suppress the kiddy monster within us and let the little angels shine through.

After breakfast we all got our coats together and got ready to go to school. All we had to do was simply walk across the street and were there. All of us would walk over together, and then separate to go to our individual classrooms. We would meet up again after school let out and walk back to Marilyn's. It became a routine that would last for several years in our lives.

That first year at Marilyn's started for my brother and I late in the school year. The school term only had a few more weeks to go until summer break. That first summer break was in fact the best summer of my early childhood. This was the first summer I would spend with friends my age having fun on the warm sunny days.

Later on Marilyn and her daughters decided to expand their daycare services. They expanded to the basement of Michelle's house, Marilyn's oldest daughter, and brought in many more children. The basement was completely set up to handle many children and had plenty of toys and activities for us to keep us from sinking into summertime boredom which would ultimately lead to mischievous behavior.

The back yard was filled with outdoor toys, and there was even a large tree with a rope hanging from it. Swinging on the rope became a right of passage to see who could swing the highest or to see who was daring enough to swing and let go just as you reached the highest point. This was the ultimate place to have fun during the summer. There were plenty of other children to play with and numerous activities in which to engage.

That summer I met several friends who remained my friends all through my elementary education. I will never forget the times I had with Tom and Gary that summer. They were the first friends I had ever made. Before them, I was never one place long enough to meet anyone or was not old enough to remember them and be able to consider them friends. I had gone through The Busy Bee in Lynchburg, The Little Buckeye in Columbus, and had not one friend to show for it. In Michelle's basement all that changed. Many long days were spent in the back yard playing with G.I. Joes or Star Wars figures in the dirt or daring each other to go yet even higher on the rope.

There were many others being cared for in the basement, but Tom and Gary became my buds. We did everything together and were saddened each evening when our parents would come to get us, knowing the day of fun was over. We would go home looking forward to the next day when everything would start all over again.

Watching us begin to make friends and beginning to settle in to our new home, invigorated Mom in her efforts at work. She saw the lights in our eyes each morning as she left us with Marilyn and knew Centerburg had become our place of security—the place we were calling home. While leaving us each morning, she noticed we had lost the fears of being left by Mom before she went to work. Before Marilyn, when she dropped us at a babysitter or in the care of daycare, she had to coax us into staying without a fountain of tears and had to reassure us she would be back to get us. Now when she left us in the care of Marilyn and her daughters she had to drag a kiss and hug from us before we happily jumped from the car and rushed into Michelle's basement.

David and I did not see this as a daycare center, but instead a place where grandma took care of us and many of our friends. This was like visiting family each day while Mom worked hard to ensure this life could be maintained or even made better. We did not have much that first year in Centerburg. Mom was running thin on resources and was not making a lot of extra money, but seeing the two of us so happy made her work to do better and to be able to offer us more.

She was going at life alone, and Marilyn gave her the opportunity to make something of herself and build something for her children.

We had now started to latch onto the kindness of this new lady and her family, and replaced the lost family members of the past with this new found family. Marilyn and her husband Merlin became our grandparents, and there two child Michelle and Marcy became our aunts. The other children being cared for replaced our cousins. We did not have any blood relation to any of these people, but David and I did not care. They were now the people who meant something to us and who were now a part of our lives. We were now from Ohio by proxy through our new family. Ohio was where we considered home, and Centerburg became our home town. We had family and friends; that was all that mattered.

16

I Received the Force

Though Dad was not spending as much time with us, he still came up at regular intervals to see us. During the summer after kindergarten, Dad came up several times. On one occasion, he took David and I out to the movies. He was only in Ohio for the weekend and did not have much time to do anything else, so the movie turned out to be a good way to spend time with his kids. I do not think he realized taking us to the movies would lead to an obsession in my life that I have even to this day.

He bought three tickets to *The Empire Strikes Back* and led us into the theater. Himself already a big fan of the *Star Wars* movies had anticipated the sequel and was eager to see it. David and I did not know much about the movie. I was not even one when the first had come out, and David was not old enough to be interested in anything more then *Peter Pan* or something of the like. I believe the only reason we even went to see *The Empire Strikes Back* was due to the fact no cartoons or any other Disney movies were playing at the time. If one had been, David and I more than likely would have demanded to see the other instead of a science fiction movie we knew little about.

After several trips to the concession stand and a trip to the bathroom, the three of us made it in to the theater and took a seat. *"In A Galaxy, Far, Far Away"* started a frenzy for me that will last the rest of my life. The movie started my first childhood obsession. I wanted everything Star Wars from that point on. The movie totally captivated my imagination. I was horrified when they froze Han Solo and fell in love with Yoda. The light sabers mystified me, and Darth Vader terrified me. This movie rocked my little world!

On the way home I made the light saber noises and howled like Chewbacca. I had chosen a career as a Jedi Knight and had the dream of one day fighting along side Luke and Yoda against the dreaded Empire. David took the movie a little different. It scared him in much the same way a horror movie would have. Darth Vader was creeping into his dreams and causing many sleepless nights.

Those two hours spent with Dad that weekend gave me a passion that later would be looked at as something only geeks were interested, but it has stuck with me. He gave me an imaginative outlet that weekend that would nurture my dreams and inspire my creativity. I now had something that made me look to the sky and to envision what was out there and how I would get there.

That same weekend, Dad took me to the toy store and bought me my first action figures and miniature ships. This would be the beginning of a collection that ended up with over eight hundred pieces by the time I entered the sixth grade. He had bought me the first pieces of a collection that would be added to with great care over my childhood, and then, even extend into adult hood as the new trilogy was released. He started a trend that would cost Mom and him thousands of dollars over the years.

Not only had I been bitten by the Star Wars bug, but many others had as well including my friends. I would not have to play alone when it came to battling the Empire. I had others who would role play with me on those hot summer days. Together, my friends and I had created an entire story line only the three of us knew about or could understand. Everyone else was standing on the outside looking in at what seemed to be random acts in the backyard. But to us, each imaginary battle was a triumph of the force over the dark side.

We were able to take the story way beyond Cloud City or the planet of Hoth into a completely new story line. We were literally acting out our own continuation of the movie. New characters were created and new adventures imagined.

David did not fall into the *Star Wars* trap. His excitement went to a new cartoon that had started to play on the after school programming. While I was fighting the evil Empire, he was fighting Skeletor and his many henchmen bent of taking over Castle Grey Skull. He-Man quickly became his childhood addiction. He dreamed of owning his very own Battle Cat or having mischievous adventures with Orco.

Before this summer, David and I shared our toys and pretty much had the same interests in what we played with in our free time. Now a line had been drawn. We did not want to play with the same old toys anymore. We had moved from the Fisher-Price toys to more grown up toys in our eyes. Stuffed animals and blocks had lost favor with the two of us. We still shared, but we had different interests; eliminating fights over toys. I did not want to play with *He-Man* action figures, and he did not want to play with my *Star Wars* ships and action figures.

The days of going into a toy store and coming out with a few toys both of us would enjoy had now faded to the past. A trip to Toys R Us now entailed getting *He-Man* and *Star Wars* at the same time. You could not buy one of us something and not the other. If David got a *He-Man* action figure, I had to get a new ship or new figure as well.

Later that summer, just before I started the first grade, the original film *Star Wars* played on television and gave me the opportunity to see the movie that had started everything. This was still before VCRs so Mom could not go to the video store and pick me up a copy—there were no video stores yet. I had to watch the movie with the occasional interruption of commercials through the bits of snow—we were to far out in the country to get cable and there was no Direct TV. The original movie only encouraged my enthusiasm for the saga that had captivated my dreams.

Unlike a couple of Christmases before, Mom and Dad would have no doubt what Santa Clause would be leaving us for the next several Christmases. The *Star Wars* and *He-Man* fascination gave them a sure thing each year. It also made birthdays and other occasions very easy to buy for. The wonder was removed. It was also very clear what gifts were for whom when Christmas rolled around or on birthdays, etc.

Like many times in life, growth is very slow most of the time, but there are instances when growth seems to happen over night. This particular summer David and I changed, matured more then we had in the few years we had been alive. We now had friends. Our taste in the toys we wanted and the play time activities had changed. Preschool past times no longer were enough to keep us occupied. Both of us were starting to talk very clearly, and we starting to comprehend more of the world around us.

Mom began to notice the breaking away of her children. We no long cried for her not to leave us; we both became less dependent on her security in a noticeable way. Her boys were still very young, but a milestone in their development was evident that summer. She could start to see what it meant to be a mother and to let go. We still needed her and her loving support, but we had started to do things on our own. Mom did not have to be everywhere we were at every moment of the day. We were no longer saddened when she left for work or had to go to school without her presence.

We were starting to understand some of life's many facts. Mom had to work, but would be back at the end of the day to get us. We had to go to school but would be going home again in the afternoon. A small piece of our innocence was left behind that summer. A small life objective had been achieved, and my brother and I were heading towards the next. Life was moving forward as it inevitably does, and all three of us were become more and more comfortable in our new home.

17

The First Few after Settling In

When I started the first grade we had been in Ohio for several years. Lynchburg was all but forgotten. Mom kept up with those in her home town via long distance telephone calls with her oldest sister and from her old friends she had worked with. But even to her, the southern ties were starting to fade. The people she had grown up with started to become distant. Lives started to grow apart. The past was the only thing they were starting to have in common. When she called home it was becoming the conversation of old friends who talked every so often to reminisce in the past and to briefly update each other how the other was doing, but really having nothing left in common.

Dad was the only person we saw from the old life. He would come to visit roughly once a month for a weekend to checkup on his two children. When he would leave, David and I had forgotten where he was going back to. We knew he was going to Virginia, but the memories of Virginia had faded. Ohio was the only home we knew anymore. Our accent had even changed to match that of those around us. We were talking true Yankee now.

Mom had done what she had set out to do. She had uprooted her family and successfully replanted it in the heart of America's bread basket. Moving to a new city in a new state and successfully becoming a part of the community was a huge obstacle on my mother's shoulders. With her hard work and with the open arms of Marilyn, she had succeeded in a way she never thought was possible. Even though she had a desire to change her life, she thought her move was going to be a failure, but it had not.

As a safety net she had kept a property in Lynchburg, rented while she was in Ohio. It was the last remaining piece of her failed marriage. With her triumph at her new job, she was now certain going back was not an option and sold that last remnant to her past. Her triumphs drove her to do even better at work.

She was now determined to break the boundaries typical of a divorced mother of two. She did not want to be a statistic of mothers barely able to keep food on the table while working two jobs. She wanted better for her two boys, and her success so far gave her the necessary courage to do what had to be done. She was going to show the world what a driven woman could do. She focused herself at Nationwide and pressed forward to further ensure the happiness of her two children.

By the time I was started the first grade, life had become a pretty nice routine for the three of us. Each morning during the week, Mom would get us up and get us to Michelle's and head into work. I would go to school with my friends during the day while David passed the daytime hours with his friends playing blissfully in the basement or out in the backyard of the daycare.

In the evenings Mom would cook something for diner. Often she would be very tired after a long day at work so she would cook something fast and easy. She never was much of a cook anyway, so anything that came out of box was a sure thing. At least it would taste alright. David and I became quite accustomed to macaroni and cheese, hotdogs, fried chicken—the simple foods really.

While dinner was cooking and she was winding down from her long day, I would play outside with David or watch television. *Star Trek* came on FOX at six, and I really liked Bones and Spock. It was a nightly routine to watch the reruns. It seemed to fit into the *Star Wars* craze I was having. Around seven each evening I had to take my nightly bath and get ready for bed at nine. Then the day would start over the next day.

During the weekends, David and I would watch cartoons; then we would have to clear the previous week's mess. Mom was too tired to clean everyday. She opted to let everything pile up during the week, and then get up late on Saturday and clean the house before the new week started. I knew I would not be allowed to go outside to play unless my room was in order. David and I would usually have to do a couple other chores before we were actually done for the day, but Mom did most everything other then cleaning our rooms.

It would still be couple more years before she would let me mow the grass. She was afraid I would hurt myself mowing the large yard with a push mower. David and I were put on weed duty pulled weeds from the flower beds and from the cracks in the sidewalk. It kept us busy, and she really was not much concerned with everything in the yard being perfect. Being out in the country, people did not care if there were weeds in your yard or if the mowing was uneven. Mom's concern was not on the small details of the home, but on her work. Often she would sit at the dining room table working with various papers in preparation for the coming work week.

When I started the second grade, David started kindergarten. With both of us in school, my brother and I started to show real individualism. Before, the only differences between the two of us were the toys we wanted, but David still did pretty much anything I did. Now he was making his own friends and was developing a personality that was all his own. Where there were once only a few differences, there were now many more and they were continuing to grow.

Our tastes in food started to separate. David liked hotdogs, and I like hamburgers. He wanted ham; I wanted turkey. David drank milk; I drink juice. Soon our refrigerator had to have two sets of foods. The foods David would eat, and the foods I would eat. Life was starting to become more complicated and more intimate between the three of us. Each of us knew what the others liked and understood the little corks each of us were starting to develop. Mom already had hers, but we had never really noticed until we started to develop our own. We had become the typical family sharing in each others lives in ways the outside world could not understand.

During the second grade, the winter brought with it far more snow then we were accustomed to. Since our time in Ohio, it had snowed during the winter months, and we had become used to the longer winter then those in Lynchburg, but we were completely surprised when the blizzard hit. Everyone seemed to talk about blizzards of the past, but this was the first we had encountered.

That winter it snowed several feet, practically burying us in our home. The roads were completely impassable, and those roads that had been plowed could only be plowed with one lane open. There was simply too much snow for the snow trucks to push off the road. With the high winds and the continual snow, it was almost a mute point to even try to plow the roads. They seemed to recover as soon as they had been dug out.

For several days we were locked in our house as we waited for the snow to stop. Schools were closed, and Mom was unable to get to work. Even if she had been able to get to work, many of her coworkers would not be there because of the snow. Everything was effectively shut down due to the snow and the wind causing snow blackouts.

When the snow did finally subside, David and I were eager to get out and play. This was the first time we had ever seen snow so deep. This was something off television, but here it was all around us. The snow was so deep in places we could not even walk through it; it would completely swallow us up. The two backdoors of our house were unable to be opened due the snow drift running down the back of the house.

The snow finally stopped long enough for the plows to get out and get to work on the daunting task of digging out the residents. We were only stuck a day before a plow truck came down our road, cutting a lifeline from our house to the outside world where we could restock food and other essentials, but many were not so lucky. Some were stuck in there homes for several days, many without power.

This harsh snow taught the three of us a great deal about the weather and how to deal with nasty consequences of lots of snow. We were fortunate Mom had gone and done her grocery shopping early so the house was stocked with food, but from this point on she always watched the news. If a major storm was approaching, she made sure she had enough to make it for a few days if we got snowed in. We also learned about frozen pipes and how to deal with them. This was the first winter where our pipes had frozen. It always takes the absence of something for us to understand its true value. Losing our water taught us how much we depended on water service.

Electricity was another issue we all had to grapple with. We were lucky this time; we only lost power for a couple of hours during the entire storm, but the implications of power loss were enough for Mom. That spring she put in a coal and wood burning stove, always making sure she had enough wood or coal to make it through a week or so without power.

After this storm, each of us knew what we had to do in the event of bad winter weather. The bathtub had to be filled with water to give us a way of flushing the toilet. There needed to be several gallons of water for cooking. The sink facets needed to be running slightly all the time to help prevent the pipes from freezing. Wood had to be brought in so we could burn it in the event of power loss. This became the routine. None of us even had to think about it; we just did it.

This first major winter storm caught my Mom off guard, but she had learned her lessons and never again did the weather worry her or David and I. It became a way of life during the winter months, and we paid no more attention to the snow, no matter how much, anymore than we did a spring shower. It became something that could be dealt with and was not a reason to panic.

18

Tootsie and Charlie

It is a right of passage for a boy to have a dog when he is growing up. Every boy should have a dog to play with and to bond with in their younger years. David and I had had a dog named Bow in Lynchburg, but we had never had a dog in Ohio. This was partly because until we planted ourselves in Centerburg, we did not live in a place where dogs were allowed. Only out in the country, with lots of places to roam, did it become just a matter of time before a dog became a part of the family.

Just a few months after moving into our house in Centerburg, Mom had taken in a dog from a coworker no longer able to care for the dog. The dog was a female German Shepard named Frauline. Frauline took to David and I immediately, but seemed to always be David's dog. She would play with me out in the yard, but when given a choice she would spend her time at David's side. She was even more protective of David then of me. When David and I would get in a fight, no matter who started the fight, Frauline would always side with David and come running to his rescue.

It did not just stop with me. One weekend when Dad was up visiting, David had decided to use the living room walls as his personal coloring book. When Dad caught him drawing his trees and giant sun on the wall he grabbed David by the arm to stop him. The wrath of our mother when she came in to see what David had done clearly rang in his mind. He would be blamed, because he had not been paying attention to what he was doing. When he grabbed David's arm, Frauline grabbed him and made it very clear, if he did not let go she was going to dig deeper and make him let go. From then on Dad had to make sure Frauline was locked in the garage or outside before he went to correct his youngest son. If David was up to his mischievous boyish ways, Frauline had to be out of the picture before he could do anything to get him to stop.

For Mom, Frauline was a way of protection. She saw the dog was extremely territorial and made her feel a little more secure at night knowing Frauline was sleeping inside the house. The dog would bark whenever something came into the yard and stood just inside the house ready when someone came to the door. She became Mom's version of a man with a baseball bat with the intention of protecting the family.

On one of Dad's weekend visits, he noticed Frauline and I were not as close and David and Frauline were. He would see me in the yard playing by myself while David and the dog frolicked in the fields, and he decided to get me a best friend to play with. His intentions were very admirable, but I am not to sure about his choice in pets for me. He came home one evening with a lamb and told me this would be my playmate. Mom even had some doubts as to the animal he decided to get his son as a pet, but the moment I saw him I loved him like nothing else in the world.

I named the lamb Tootsie, and we became best friends. David had his dog, and I had my lamb. Tootsie took to life at our house with zeal. Unlike the dog, Tootsie was not allowed in the house, but there was a fenced in area in the back with a small sheltered area made of blue tarp that suited him just fine. Each day before going to school I would take food out and put it in Tootsie's food dish. In the evenings I would let the lamb out of the fenced area, and we would play in the yard. Tootsie never left the yard. He never really went more then ten feet from me. As I played in the dirt with my Star Wars figures, Tootsie would be right there eating grass or trying to eat my toys.

Late in August a nasty storm came up quick and the high winds blew Tootsie's little shed of tarp across the yard. Seeing the lamb crying in the storm, Mom and I went out and took him to a small shed at the back of our property. It was not the best shed in the world, but it would serve its purpose for the evening and keep the lamb out of the weather for the night. We made sure he was locked in good and rushed back to the house through the pouring rain and howling winds.

The next morning we woke up with the power out. Mom opened the windows to let the air blow through the house to keep it cool and made cereal for David and I. After breakfast David and Frauline went out to play, and I went to the shed to get Tootsie. It had been a long night, and I was sure he was scared after the storm. When I got to the shed the door was open slightly, and I was worried he had got out during the night, but was relieved when I saw him lying in the corner. I pulled the door fully open and called his name, but he did not move. I went up to his side and gently shook him to wake him up, but when I pulled my hands away they were covered in blood. I touched the little lamb again to make sure he was not just sleeping.

With blood running through my fingers, I ran back to the house, eyes full of tears and told Mom Tootsie was hurt and needed help. Seeing my hands, Mom jumped into a panic and asked me where I was hurt. She was not listening to me. It was not mine; it was my lamb's. It took a few minutes and a good rinsing in the kitchen sink for her to listen to what I was saying. She had to make sure my hands were not hurt before she would come with me.

It was obvious to Mom that during the night a dog or something had killed my lamb. Since the shed was so far away we were unable to hear Tootsie's cries for help during the night. Mom took on the job of burying my pet, and then offering her comfort to me. I cried for several hours that day and was glum for several weeks after his death. I loved that lamb; now he was gone, and I was left to play alone again.

Entering the third grade that fall took my mind off the loss of my lamb, but I never really forgot him. Seeing me play in the backyard alone again, Dad decided to get me another friend. He could not bear to see his son so unhappy and was determined to do whatever it took to make me smile again. Dad had not been here when Tootsie died, but he felt responsible for my pain because he had brought him home. To make amends for the loss and to help me move forward, he took me to the dog pond in Mount Vernon and told me to pick my dog. He gave me the option of any dog in the pound.

I walked up and down the rows of cages and looked in at everyone they had. Each one was perfect in their own way. Each of them came up and licked my hands through their cages and barked to get my attention. They all knew I was there to take one of them home. They had been through the routine before. After a good period of time, Dad asked if there was one I wanted, and I told him I wanted them all. Dad would have taken them all for me if he did not fear the wrath of an angry ex-wife as he brought a truck load of dogs home.

He told me to keep looking until I could settle on one. After several more minutes, I choose the dog looking like a mix between a Lab and Beagle. His name was Charlie, and he was still just a puppy. Before I could change my mind, Dad had the attendant take Charlie out of his cage and brought him up front away from the other dogs. After signing a few papers Dad loaded the two of us into his Chevet, and we headed back home.

Charlie was full of life and was every kid's dream of a dog. He liked to play, and he was all mine. He was attached to me from the very moment he was taken out of his cage. This was my dog and would become my new friend.

When we got home, Mom watched as I brought my new friend into the house. She was happy to see me so happy again but was not sure a new pet was something she wanted to take on. She had just eased me through the death of one and did not want to see that happen again. She also was not sure Charlie would have been a great choice in dogs. Charlie was wild; it was obvious from the moment we got out of the car.

He was not mean, but he ran wide open all the time. This was a kid's dog but not really a house friendly dog. After a few weeks, I ended up having to keep him outside when we were not home. Charlie would rip the curtains from the windows, tear up the cushions on the sofa, and string trash through out the house. He just wanted to play all the time. When he was left alone with no one to keep him company, he would make up other things to occupy his time. These other activities usually entailed destroying something in the house.

Mom would get so mad when she came home to a house torn up by the dog. She would yell at Charlie for doing wrong and then yell at Frauline for letting Charlie do all his destructive actions. But as soon as I came in and hugged Charlie, letting him know I still loved him, Mom would back off. I would have to clean up the mess, but she would suppress her anger when she saw how happy I was with him.

When we started leaving him outside, he would dig up Mom flower gardens in protest and string paper and toys throughout the yard. He was just the same whether in the house or outside. To try to stop him from getting into so much trouble, Mom made me chain him up at the corner of the house before we left. When we did that he simply started to rip the siding off the house and chew it into small pieces. The white flecks of plastic would be everywhere when we got home.

While home, I insisted the dog be allowed inside. Frauline was allowed in the house, so Charlie must also be in the house, at least when I am home. With the two of us in the house, Mom seemed to always be yelling at the two of us to stop running, stop jumping around, and to go outside and play. As it got colder and colder outside, we started playing more and more in the house. After pulling out most of her hair and as she put it, "I have had it up to here with you and Charlie," Mom decided it was time for Charlie to go.

It was getting close to Thanksgiving and Dad had come up a week before the holiday and was due to stay a week after the holiday since we had extra time off from school. After a couple of days of being around Charlie and I, he started to understand the frustrations Mom was having with the two of us. He agreed with her; Charlie had to go. Since Dad had given me the dog, Mom gave him the job of taking the dog away. Neither really knew how to do this. They saw the two of us together and knew I would be devastated if I had to give away my dog and would never let them do it. I would not let him go.

The night after Thanksgiving, I put Charlie out in the garage so he would not root through the trash or tear up the living room while I slept. I left him with the expectation of seeing him in the morning, but when I woke up and went to feed him, Charlie was gone. The door to the garage was open and my dog was gone. It was not to long ago that I lost Tootsie, now I lost Charlie. Mom and Dad gave me many hugs while a cried having lost my dog. I spent all day looking for him. I even had Dad drive me up and down the streets looking for him. I wanted him back so bad. I could not figure out what I had done to make him run away. Even if the door was opened, he knew where he lived and always came back. But this time he never did.

That night Dad kept me company as I cried myself to sleep. Mom even tried to comfort me by telling me Charlie may have went to a family who needed him more then we did. It was so upsetting, and it was not until the Christmas holiday rolled around that I started to forget about Charlie and how he had left me—how my best friend deserted me that night.

I was twenty-two when I learned what really happened to Charlie that night. Dad and I were talking and some how the dogs of my past came up in conversation, and I spoke about Charlie. I had many dogs after Charlie, but I never forgot about him. I talked about how I still wondered what had happened to him, and Dad was shocked that I did not know. He figured Mom would have told me by now. I told him I had no idea, and he finally let me know what happened to my fury childhood friend.

After I had gone to sleep that night, Dad loaded Charlie into his car and drove him to Mount Vernon back to the pound. Since it was late at night and a holiday weekend the pound was not open; so Dad took Charlie out of the car and placed an open bag of dog food in front of the door to the pound and left Charlie. He drove off after leaving my dog in the cold to fend for himself until someone either took him home or put him back into the pound.

Both Mom and Dad were in on this plan. They figured, if they left the door open they would be able to convince me Charlie had run away, and it worked. Even though they had everything figured out, as soon as Dad got home, Mom told him to go back and get Charlie. Dad did not hesitate. He simply backed back into the road and again headed to Mount Vernon. He had the long ride home to think about what he done and she was looking at me sleep, knowing I was going to be very hurt when I got up in the morning. Though Charlie was a nuisance to Mom and Dad, I loved him and, therefore, he was a part of the family.

As Dad approached the pound for the second time that night, he saw Charlie lying in the road. A car had hit and killed him while he wandered in the cold dark. He put Charlie's body in the backseat of the car and drove back to Centerburg. Dad said Mom actually cried when she saw Charlie's dead body out of guilt for what they had done. Dad was given the task of going out back and burying my friend before I got up. Now they had no other choice but to tell me he had run away. I would not have been able to handle the truth. A runaway would be far easier then another death.

When Dad told me this I was not mad. It was good to know what happened, but I wasn't upset. When I think back, I am actually surprised I was able to keep the dog as long as I did. He was a little monster and torn up more stuff than any other dog we had ever had. I found it more interesting that the two of them had come up with a perfect plan and then tried to back out of it. I think it actually hurt them more then it did me. They knew the tears I shed for my missing friend was because of what they had intentionally done, and because of their actions, Charlie would never come home to me even if they wanted him to.

19

Charlotte Travels with Her Job

All the while David and I are in school and making new friends, Mom was working feverishly to succeed at Nationwide. She worked many overtime hours and took on addition work related projects to help further her career. All of this hard work and many long days at the office led to several promotions. While David and I were still in the first few years of grade school, she took a position that required her to travel extensively out west. She and a group of her co-workers started setting up offices for Nationwide west of the Mississippi. This took her to Dallas, Portland, and Los Angeles to name a few.

Often she would have to leave home for weeks at a time while she did her work out west. She started out having Dad come up and watch us during the extended stays, but soon opted out of that option. She did not want her ex-husband around her new home or her two children that often. Marilyn was the next best thing. Marilyn took us in for those weeks when Mom was gone and treated us just like her own daughters.

By this time Michelle was no longer watching children in her basement, so the babysitting routine had moved back to Marilyn's house. This meant, every morning when David and I got up to great the world, a group of our friends was already there and waiting. To us these extended stays were just long sleepovers with our friends at grandma's house.

Marilyn would take us to the airport to see Mom off. We would give her hugs and kisses just before she boarded the plane; then watch through the giant glass windows until take off. The first few times were hard. Being left at a babysitter for the day was easier then being left for a couple of weeks, but eventually it became routine. David and I would watch the United Airline take to the air, then leave the airport with Marilyn.

We would all return to the airport when she returned to pick her up. After some long hugs, David and I would insist on seeing what she brought us. It never failed that on each trip she took, she returned with a bag full of things she had gathered on her travels. On one of her many trips to Portland, she brought home giant pine cones. They were almost a foot long with a diameter of six inches or so. They were huge, and there size only was enhanced as two small boys held them in their tiny hands.

She had picked the pinecones up off the ground while she was visiting Lake Tahoe on a ski trip. She told us the pinecones would freeze in the huge trees and fall to the ground like bowling balls from the sky. I could image an ice logged cone this size would fall with a huge crash, and God help anyone standing under one at the time.

As she continued to travel, she always thought of David and I. She wanted us at her side, but knew we were in school and needed to stay in Centerburg with our friends. When we were out of school for the summer, she made arrangements for us to travel with her or to at least come and visit for a few weeks. She would have to invite Dad, but to her, putting up with him was worth the opportunity to see her two boys. We were the reminder as to why she was working so hard.

Our first trip would be to Dallas, Texas. She had been there for a few weeks, and once we were out of school, she made arrangements to get us there for vacation. Dad came and got us, and we went back to Lynchburg for a few days so he could get his things together. Then the three of us headed south in Dad's Chevette. David and I had just endured the trip from Centerburg to Lynchburg—eight long hours through the mountains in the early summer without air conditioning. Now we would have to pile back into the tiny car and head out for an even longer drive.

It took Dad two days to drive from Lynchburg to Dallas. He probably could have made it in one day. He seemed to have this ability to drive for long periods of time without sleep or without stopping, but he had David and I to contend with. We had to stop frequently for bathroom breaks and were always hungry or thirsty or just wanted to get out of the car for a while. Dad tried to get us to sleep, but the long drive and with each other to pick on during the drive, there was very little sleeping happening.

Frustrated with the two of us, Dad stopped in Mississippi for the night. He had tired of breaking up backseat fights and was tired of stopping so often to help break up the monotony. He finally gave in when he knew there was not going to be any way for him to drive straight through, and checked us into a hotel. David and I were extremely relieved and immediately headed for the pool. The heat was intense, and we had been cooped up for over twelve hours. The pool became our release.

Dinner were simple Happy Meals from McDonald's, and my brother and I quickly fell asleep for the night—the air conditioning cranked so high the windows of the room frosted over during the night. Early the next morning, back in the car we went. Our next stop was Dallas, Texas.

In Dad's little car we pulled into the parking lot of one of the largest and most prestigious hotels of Dallas. It was more luxurious then many hotels designed as a resort or grand vacation get aways. The lobby was huge and filled with swanky furniture and high polished wood. Dad went up to the counter, got Mom's room number. It took as a few minutes to get through the atrium. The roof was over twelve stories above us. There was a large pool with an island, work out facilities, a restaurant, and several bars. The interior of the hotel was its own little community in itself.

Mom greeted us with her hugs and many kisses and immediately took us to the pool. We had been in a hot car for the entire day, and she new a good dip would be the thing that would sooth the traveling woes. It also gave Dad a moment to himself. After being locked in a car with two rambunxious sons, he needed a bit of a break.

We spend a couple of weeks with Mom. She would go to work during the day, and Dad would take us out to see the area or simply watch us play in the hotel until Mom got off from work. In the evenings and on the weekends, all of us would go out and experience the attractions of Texas.

Though we went to many restaurants, to a couple water parks and an amusement park, I remember the trip to Sesame Street like it was yesterday. I was able to sit on the steps next to Oscar the Grouch's trash can and was able to wonder through Mr. Cooper's store. It was exactly like I had been watching on television for years. Everything was exactly were it was supposed to be. I even was able to meet Big Bird, eat cookies with Cookie Monster, and counted with the Count.

I also went to see my first rodeo, Texas style. I have seen rodeos since this first one in Texas, but no one does it like the cowboys state does. I even got to have my own dual with a cowboy as we watched the bulls bucking their riders into the dirt while the clowns ran wildly throughout the arena.

After several more days of play in the Lone Star state, Dad loaded us back in the car and we headed for home. Mom still had a couple more weeks before she would be done, but our visit had made her time away from home a little easier. David and I picked up a plethora of stories to tell our friends when we got back home.

After several trips to Texas for work, Mom was finally finished and Nationwide was sending her to a new location. This time she would be going even further west. Los Angels, California became her new location of off site work. Again she made arrangements for my brother and I to join her while she worked. This time she planned the trip a little more precisely. The trip to Texas was spur of the moment, and things were done as they came up, not too much planning. Mom felt we wasted a lot of time at the hotel or driving to places. When she took us to California, she wanted to make sure everything was planned out, and we would be able to see everything southern California had to offer.

Instead of going out to California and then having us come in later she decided to just take us with her when she went. She made sure Dad would be coming as well. Even though she could hardly tolerate having him around most of the time, she took great solace in knowing he would be there to watch her two sons while she worked. He really was the key to being able to bring David and I with her. She would not have been able to do it without his help.

Dad had learned his lesson during the drive to Texas. There was no way he was going to drive us all the way across the country. He would loose his mind before he made it to Vegas. Flying was out due to the cost; so another way had to be found. Mom talked to a couple of her co-workers in Columbus who had made the trip before and asked how they had crossed the country. Other then flying, there was Amtrak. Nationwide used trains to move workers who were afraid of flying or had the extra day to travel and just wanted to relax for a few days.

It did not take much to convince her, a train was the way to go. It was cheap, and it was not as cramped as a car would be. Several of her fellow co-workers were also going to travel by train, giving her and Dad some company on the trip. With her travel means arranged she got all of us ready for the trip.

The train left Wooster, Ohio, around four in the morning. We boarded, and thankfully to our parents, David and I fell right to sleep with the gentle rocking of the train. Mom and Dad had everything packed and had woken us up at the very last minute to leave to catch the train. Like most little kids, when we were up, we were wide awake. During the drive to the station and while we waited for the train, both David and I could hardly contain our excitement. This led to us bouncing around in the car and aimlessly exploring the train station. Mom and Dad had been up most of the night and did not have the energy to keep up with two young boys, but they signed a thankful sigh of relief when we fell right asleep on the train.

When we awoke, we were just heading into Chicago. We had a layover and a train switch there and was able to walk around the city for a couple of hours before reboarding. Mom had packed everything we would need for the trip before we left Centerburg, but she did not understand that once the luggage was loaded into the train, she would not be able to get to them until we reached our final destination in Los Angels. That meant we did not have any change of cloths or any of the snacks she had packed. Consequently, those few hours in Chicago were mainly spent buying a few days worth of cloths and personal necessities for the trip.

We were able to go up the Sears Tower and look out through the observation deck at the sprawling city before heading back to the train station. After a few confusing minutes we found the train heading to L.A. and boarded. This would be the train that would take us to the land of Hollywood and the home of Mickey Mouse. We were in for a train ride lasting two days through the very heart of western America.

Unlike the trip to Texas, when we arrived in Los Angels, we all were full of energy and ready to get out and see the city. The train had had an observation car, several dining cars, and an entertainment car, so none of us were haggard by the long trip. We traveled in a moving hotel, where we received plenty of rest and had plenty of activities to keep boredom from creeping its way in.

Again, Nationwide did not skimp on the hotel. It was another five star establishment even grander than the one in Texas. David and I were becoming accustomed to luxurious hotels. Before these trips our only experience with a hotel had been when we first moved to Ohio. Those were memories of being cramped and nothing to do. These hotels were large and full of things to pass the time.

I had just finished the third grade that spring and was thrilled at seeing Hollywood. While Mom was working during the day, Dad would take David and I out and the first place I wanted to go was to Hollywood. I wanted to see the mountain with the giant letters planted on its side. I wanted to see the Chinese Theater with the concrete imprints of feet and hands of Hollywood's best.

Mom made sure we spent a day at Disney Land. No trip to California is complete without stopping to say hello to Mickey and his friends. We were able to ride the tea cups and had the mouse ears made with our names stitched across the front—a must have when visiting the happiest place on Earth.

Dad took the two of us to the beach several times. He would watch the woman while David and I played in the waves and built monuments in the sand. I was then able to say I had spent time in both the Atlantic and Pacific oceans. We were even able to see the place where the beach scenes of The Karate Kid were filmed—a big movie for David and I at the time, almost as big as E.T.

My time spent in Los Angels was the first family vacation I can remember and hope to be able to do again sometime. Though Mom was working, it was still a vacation for me and in most cases for her as well. She went to many of the sites and vacations spots Dad, David, and I were able to visit. We spent several weeks in California and looked forward to the next trip we would be taking wherever that may be.

Nationwide opened the world up to my family and let us enjoy the pleasures of the places they sent my mother. This insurance company and its people became a major player in the lives of David and I. The men and women my mother worked for became her family and gave her a home substitute to that in which she had left. They also gave David and I a place in Ohio.

After the trip to Los Angels, Mom went to Portland on many occasions, but was never able to get David and I out there to see her while she worked. By the time she had been able to make arrangements to get us out to the land of huge trees and great skiing, she took another position within the company. She moved up several rungs in the corporate latter. She did this partly because of the opportunity. It meant more money and more benefits, but she also did it to provide a more stable work schedule for herself. Though she was able to take us at times with her when she traveled, there were many more times when she had to leave David and I behind.

Marilyn was a wonderful person to leave her children with, but she did not want to be on the road while we were growing up. She wanted to be there to experience the little things in our lives that meant so much to us. She wanted to be there as our baby teeth fell out. She wanted to be there for the school plays and for after school sports. This new job allowed her to do that. I was getting ready to enter the fifth grade and David was not too far behind me. She would travel a little after taking the new position, but no where near as often and for much shorter periods of time. Instead of being gone for weeks at a time, she would only be gone for a few weekends of the year.

20

Innocence Lost

The year I entered the fifth grade, I switched from seeing the world through the eyes of a child and started to see the world through young adult eyes. This was a year of holding on to some of my childhood things in one hand while reaching for more adult things in the other. This year was the beginning of young adulthood. I was not quite a teenager but finally my teens were in sight. I was becoming the big boy every little kid looks forward to as they struggle to grow up in an adult world, always wanting to do what the grown ups can do.

The Christmas before had exposed Santa Clause as Mom and Dad. The tooth fairy mystery was unraveled; I simply gave the teeth to Mom and asked for the cash to buy a new Star Wars figure. The Easter Bunny was replaced by a ride to the store where I could pick out the candy I wanted instead of getting a basket full of Peeps I would eventually through away or use in my sling shot to shoot birds perched on the power line running in front of the house.

The previous years had been filled with Sesame Street, Mr. Rodgers Neighborhood, and various cartoons. Music was not existent; I know I listened to the radio, but never gave much thought to the singers. E.T. had made me cry. The Ghostbusters had made me laugh. I had watched with stun shock in the school cafeteria as the shuttle Challenger blew up in mid flight. Reagan had started to win the arms race, and Mom was glued to the television watching Oliver North answer each question "I do not recall."

With the start of this new school year, my tastes in life changed. Things that I would have never considered before started to become interesting. My life took a one eighty in the span of nine months. Life no longer was child's play but had become more serious and less playful. The blinders were starting to be lifted. I found once I started to see I could never go back. I would no longer be able to believe the childhood fantasies once I knew the truth. No longer could I go back and have those moments of pure happiness only a child could have living in a fantasy world filled with mystery created by my parents.

Unlike the past, music started to become an important past time. No longer did the child sing-a-longs of the past meet my musical tastes. Bon Jovi and AC/DC had moved in. Michael Jackson came into favor with his Bad album. Though I had seen thriller many times before, he now was considered cool to listen too, and I understood why he was cool to listen to.

With VCRs now in almost every home, the movies of the past were out. No longer did I seek to see the latest animated flick from Disney; I wanted to see movies about aliens and monsters crawling in the night. I was no longer afraid of the man in the hockey mask or the man with knives for fingers. I wanted to see what the adults were watching. I did not want to see cartoons with flying boys or kissing dogs.

The *Cat In The Hat* did not nurture my fantasies anymore. I no longer needed books with lots of pictures or pop up cardboard scenes. Books with lots of words were coming into favor. I had collections now, not toys. The Star War action figures and models I played with were no longer things to play with but things to collect. Playing in the play ground at recess became kick ball or softball. The swings and monkey bars began to loose there childhood wonder and excitement.

School itself took on a new life. Before, school had been something to do during the day in order to spend time with friends. Getting good grades had never been at the top of my list of things to do when in school. But now grades started to matter. It became a challenge to see how well I could do. I had not been a bad student, but I had not been a good student academically. Now it was time to change all that. I wanted to get my tests back with as many questions right as possible. I wanted to spell every word correctly on spelling tests. I wanted to do better then what I had been doing. At the time I had not seen the significance of doing well, but I wanted to see the good grades. It was a game to me. The better the grade, the more I was winning.

Mrs. Holly, my fifth grade teacher was the teacher who really brought out or at least demanded my best. She saw I could do better and made me do it. I was not able to slide by in her class. She made it to where I had to study to do better. Though she was tough, she started my study and reading skills. I did average in her class, but she pushed me in the right direction with my studies. She showed me the importance of reading and diligently studying to make good grades. It would take me a couple of years to polish my reading and study skills, but when I did, the world of academics opened up to me. She pushed me into becoming a good student later in my life when my life actually depended on the grades I made.

In Mrs. Holly's class I was brought back in touch with an old friend from the first grade. Jason and I had been friends off and on through out the years but from this point on we would be friends all the way through high school and even after. Though we did not always remain close friends, we were always a part of each other's lives. Our paths were always close to each other. Jason became one of those few people who remain in my life regardless of how I changed or how he changed as we entered and exited our teenage years.

This year in school also introduced me to the ladies in a new way. I had had several girlfriends before the fifth grade. We would sit together at lunch and hang out on the play ground during recess. I even received my first kiss by the swing set. But now sex education opened my eyes to ladies. I now saw them in a different way. The potential to have fun with the ladies became more than a kiss on the play ground or someone to have lunch with.

My best friend from the past Gary faded away to a new set of friends. These new friends would be my best buds until I entered high school in a few years. These friends were the transition friends from childhood to young adulthood. Though the bonds between us would not last, they were strong none the less. Jason would be the only one to make it through the many years until graduation and then after high school.

For Mom this year was the year she saw her little boy become a little man. My wants started to change and my privacy was important to me. She looked at me and saw the beginning of the end of my innocence and blissful days as a child. She started to see how the world would soon start to put its weight on my shoulders. The pressures of adulthood would soon be upon me, and she did everything to further extend the fantasy world without cares.

That summer Mom planned a trip to Florida. Disney World being the actual destination, I insisted on going to Cape Canaveral. I wanted to see NASA. Mickey and Tinkerbell no longer interested me. I wanted to see the rocket ships and dreamed of being an astronaut. I was beginning to understand the sacrifice made at the Apollo One launch site dedicated to those who burned in the tragedy. I looked at the launch pad with wonder and a dream of one day going into space myself.

My career dreams would change over the years, but I no longer wanted to be a super hero or a cowboy. My sites had turned to a dream which, with effort, could be made into reality. I still held onto the joys of the Disney theme park, but instead of seeking the fairy tales of The Magic Kingdom, I sought the wonders of Epcot Center. This vacation was the last vacation where I was a little boy in a world of dreams. From here on out vacations would be different. I would seek the beach and the ladies in bikinis over the Pixie Dust vacations of the past.

21

My First Steps to Adulthood

By the end of the sixth grade, everything about the previous twelve years of my life had changed. My bed room, with its Looney Tune wallpaper and Star Wars curtain and bed spread to match, was all redone. I now had the room of a man. I threw out the t-shirts with Yoda or Darth Vader on them and replaced them with a more stylish grown up look. Instead of wearing jeans and athletic shoes all the time, I now mixed things up with dress shoes and khaki pants.

The person who had existed just a few years earlier had been replaced by a boy getting ready to take his first steps into adulthood. With the sixth grade behind me, high school was ahead of me. I was going to be going to school in the building that as a kindergartner terrified me. It would soon become my school time home, and I would look at it as a place of happiness and many wonderful memories.

Centerburg did not really have a middle school when I entered the seventh grade. Everyone was in elementary until the sixth grade and from seven through twelve was considered high school. Centerburg was not large enough to have a middle school all to its own. Before leaving elementary school, I was introduced to the high school life through a sit in program. This was an attempt to ease the transition between the one room teaching environments to the multi-classroom environment.

Even with all the efforts by the teachers, everyone going to the high school for the first time were nervous and not really sure about what it would be like or even what to expect when they got there, myself included. The summer before Dad came and took David and I for the summer. We spend a lazy summer in Lynchburg, getting up late, fishing, and doing nothing that really required any kind of work.

During the summer, each Saturday we would go to the flea market to hunt for deals. Dad was still looking for all kinds of car parts and body parts to further his work rebuilding cars. Just like when Mom and him were married, his house was filled with oily parts and his back yard had piles a rusting metal he swore he would fix and make money. While on one of our trips to the flea market, I saw a book titled *Pet Sematary* by an author I had heard about but never read. Until now I was not really interested in reading a book quite this long. But I had seen the movie and wondered what the book would be like.

It took me just a week to read the entire book, and I was hooked on Stephen King. Each Saturday I sought out anything written by him or any author that wrote in the horror genre. Digging through the boxes of books and asking the various people selling their books, I was introduced to Dean Koontz, Clive Barker, Michael Crichton, and many more. I fell in love with the horror stories I was reading.

Before then, horror and science fiction had been an obsession of mine, but never before had I had started to read into the genres. My reading skills before the sixth grade really did not give me the opportunity to experience the magic of these books. Now with the reading and comprehension skills needed to enjoy these books, I could not get my hands on enough of them. They became a way for me to leave the world and enter into another one. They were also a way for me to forget the worries of starting high school in the fall. These books became the place I could go to forget about the world around me.

When the summer was over and Dad brought David and I back to Ohio, I had over two hundred books dealing in everything from slimy, slithery beasts to aliens from far away worlds. I had a collection of over two hundred worlds that would be my escape when the worries of school started to lay heavy on my mind.

When it was time to start school, instead of going to Marilyn's each morning with Mom, David and I would now catch the bus. I was a big boy and did not need a babysitter anymore. I could catch the bus in the morning and come home in the evening on the bus. It was only a couple of hours when Mom would not be there watching me, and the neighbors were not to far if I needed something.

With hesitation she conceded to letting me get on the bus in the morning and come home on the bus. She did this with the threats of taking me back to Marilyn's if I missed the bus, did anything to David, or just did anything she did not like. With the fear of having to go back to the babysitter, I made sure I did not screw up. It was not that I did not like Marilyn; she was a part of my family. I had known her longer then any other person in Ohio, other than Lori and her family. I just did not want to have to tell people I had to go to a babysitter because my mother did not think I was able to stay at home for a few hours.

A few days before school started I went to the school and got my schedule and locker assignment. I walked the halls looking for the classes so I would have some idea where I would be going when it actually came time to start school. I had been given a tour of the high school before the end of the previous school year, but I could not remember a thing. I made sure I knew where the bathrooms were and where I would have to go for study hall, gym, and each of my other classes.

Mom had already bought everything I would need to get started. All that was left to do was to wait and to think about the approaching day. Dad had gone back to Lynchburg, and I was left at a house in the country to worry about the many imaginary dilemmas and nightmares that may lie ahead of me that first day. Almost everything I could conceive was far worse than anything that could actually happen and I knew it. But once the ideas had crept their way into my head, they would not leave. They only grew and got worse with each devious growth spurt.

Mom did what she could to calm my nerves. She told me not to concern myself with what was going to happen at school. She told me just after a week of school starting, the old building in which the high school resided would feel like home, and the comforting halls of the elementary would seem like the distant past. When that did not work, she sent me outside to mow the lawn. Mowing would either take my mind off school or wear me out, and I would be able to sleep well that night.

Mowing the lawn had been given over to David and I a couple years back, when Mom finally sprung for riding lawn mower. Now yard work became a way for her to keep us busy. With so much yard and so many trees and bushes in the yard to weed around, I would be busy almost a good weekend to get everything done. That weekend before high school started, I mowed the grass and forgot for a moment what was coming up, just as she had hoped it would. It took me the entire weekend to finish all the trim and weeding. Before I knew it, Monday rolled around—the first day.

When the big day finally came around, I reluctantly got on the bus and headed to the beginning of young adulthood. With that first step onto the bus, everything I was as a child changed—lost to memories and the past. Where I was once holding on to things of the past in one hand while reaching towards adulthood with the other, I was now letting go of the things and with both hands was grabbing for the person I would become for the rest of my life. I still had a great ways to go before I would have an identity that would stick, but my arms were now open, free to embrace the future that now lay ahead of me.

After a half hour of riding on the bumpy bus, I was finally there for the first day of school. I got off the bus and headed into the large building amidst people who where a lot taller and bigger than me and waded through to my locker. With my coat put away, I went to my first class—pen and paper in hand, nervous enough to be sweating through the palms of my hands, legs weak with anticipation.

I sat down and looked at the other people in my class. These were all people I had went through grade school with, but none of us really said a word to each other. Everyone had the same stares of panic and fear as we waited for the class to begin.

No one knew what to expect next. Only one thing was for certain. Whatever was going to happen would happen to us all. We would all be going through this together. Each of us had made those first steps that morning, whether it was getting on the bus, walking, or catching a ride with parents. Yesterday was the last day of childhood. This was the first day in a long run of many days—some good, some bad, that would lead us into the world of the adults.

22

The Early High School Years

It took a few days to get used to the new high school, but just like Mom had said, after a week, I felt right at home. The elementary school just across the field was a past I could never recover and had no desire to ever go back.

It took a while to get used to getting from one class to another without being late. With my locker on the third floor, getting where I needed to go before the bell rang was not a problem unless my class was on the first floor. Running through the hoards of people to my locker and then back to class on the first floor was like fighting an uphill avalanche of people.

It really was not a problem, if I was going to gym or art class. The teachers of those classes rarely noticed if you were a few seconds late. Study Hall was the class I had to worry about. Located in the basement, it would take everything I had in me to get there on time each day. But there were occasions when I did not make. Mr. Nixon, the babysitter while the students pretended to be working on something of value, hated two things—those who talked and those who were late.

Mr. Nixon was the shop teacher, but on his off period he would sit in and make sure study hall ran smoothly. Instead of sitting at the desk like most normal teachers, he put a student desk on top of the teacher's desk so he could see everyone in the class and glare at them with his piercing stare. He was the big scary man sitting up high looking down at his little minions. If that was not bad enough, he had an interesting way of dealing with people who were late or decided to break the dead silence with a word or some laughter.

The room was in the basement and at one time was a small gym with a small stage at one end. The ceiling was at least twenty feet overhead and the floor and walls were made of concrete and cinderblock. The old stage had been filled in with a wall, painted with a giant picture of a sun smiling down on the students. It looked very similar to the sun from the old Raisin Brand cereal commercials assuring everyone there were two scoops of raisins in every box. The sun came be know as Mr. Sunshine with Mr. Nixon.

If you were caught talking or came in just a hair past the ringing of the starting bell, he would make you talk to Mr. Sunshine through the entire study hall period. The tardy students or those who could not keep their mouths shut would have to stand for the forty minute class and talk to the painting like it was a person for all to hear. Of course the rest of us had to do everything in our power not to snicker or laugh at those talking to Mr. Sunshine. We did not want to have to talk to the wall all period.

Most of the conversations to Mr. Sunshine were very light. The students would try to get others in the class to laugh so they would have some company while talking to the wall. One student even talked about Mr. Nixon to Mr. Sunshine. That turned out to be a very interesting conversation to listen in on. Mr. Nixon even allowed the student to talk the entire week to Mr. Sunshine to get everything off his chest.

I was able to avoid talking to the wall for several weeks, before eventually time caught up with me, and I was talking to the wall. I ended up having to talk to Mr. Sunshine a couple of times that year, before I completely got the hang of getting to class on time. Later I would come to like Mr. Nixon. After taking his shop class, I was able to see he was a great teacher and no where near as scary as I had first thought him to be. When David finally made it into high school, Mr. Nixon would become his favorite teacher, talking fondly about him even to this day.

Mr. Davis opened my eyes to math the first few years of high school. Until I was taught under him, my math skills were lacking, and it was not a class I really wanted to have a part in, but he stuck with me. He also turned out to be one of the most off beat teachers I would know with his wild antics and dry humor. Between him and Mr. Madza, the art teacher, I had two teachers who had a hippie demeanor with a way of carrying themselves that just made you laugh and feel comfortable when around them.

Mrs. Huddleston was my English teacher, and she introduced me to the red pen, forcing perfection out of each of her students. Before her, I saw few red marks on papers I wrote or assignments I completed. With her, I think she used an entire pen just to grade my work. I would get back assignments with so much red on them I could not make out my original work.

There were many other teachers, each of them giving a piece of themselves to each student they taught. Each class had a different aurora about it. Rules were different from teacher to teacher, and I had to learn what I could get away with in each class based on the one teaching the class. Just like people, each class had its own personality. If you did not like the class of straight teaching, all you had to do was just wait. The next class was sure to be different.

Though the seventh and eighth grades were exciting times for me, the really fun times would not come until the ninth grade. In these early years, our classes were very similar to that in elementary; we just moved from room to room with each subject. Classes were already determined. In the ninth grade, I would be able to choose what I wanted to get involved in and what classes I wanted to take. These first few years were just a transition from the old to the new. This was the opportunity to be exposed to different avenues of study and the many teachers and teaching styles. Very soon I would have some control over what I learned and would start to be given the wheel to my life.

This mix of teachers gave all of us the ability to learn in different ways. Some teachers taught through a book and notes, while others taught with a hands on approach. Some encouraged creativity over perfection, while others scrutinized each letter or number of an assignment for errors. This mix encouraged everyone to try different approaches at learning. I learn very well from reading a book and taking notes. I am also more creative than a perfectionist, but with this variety of teaching styles, I learned many different ways to learn.

I have found that being creative works well when I am working on a marketing campaign, but perfection is required to gather demographics for a specific project. These various ways of accomplishing the tasks put before me were learned in the early years of high school. They have been refined over the years, but it all started with the mixture of teaching styles I encountered in the seventh grade.

I may have struggled with my studies for a while, but I was learning something more important. The world does not always want someone who is creative or book smart. The adult world requires a blend of creativity, with perfection, while working both in the field and back at the office. By adapting to the ways I was being taught, I was picking up a versatility skill essential later in life.

Getting accustomed to the new way of school was only part of the first few years in high school. New friends were made and old ones were lost. These years were the years I would grow the most—almost a foot and half in two years. Everything was changing in irreversible ways as I moved along life towards adulthood. I once looked just beyond the horizon and saw high school and getting my drivers license. I now looked and saw graduation and college. As the weeks went by life seemed to speed up with each passing day. Not quite in the driver's seat of my future, I looked ahead and wondered what it would be like, what I would be doing, and who I would meet.

The world was now becoming the world of opportunities, no longer the world of fantasies. It was an exciting time, when anything could happen. I was only limited by the roof I put over my imagination and dreams. I no longer saw the world as a land a fairytales created by my parents, but I was now starting to see the reality of life. I was still looking through the protective lens Mom had put up to protect me from the full harshness of the outside world, but it was more real then anything I had seen before.

By the end of the seventh grade, the eighties had ended, George Bush was in the White House, and the Berlin wall had crumbled. I had started with records, moved to cassette tapes and was now listening to compact disks. Michael Jackson had officially become a white guy, and rap was becoming the music of choice. The nineties were here and would take me into my adult life. I finally began my teen years and was counting down until I could drive. The move from the Centerburg elementary school to the high school was a move from the past to the future. Life would not change as drastically for me until graduation and the beginning of college.

23

Mom Turned Back

My first year of high school was a turning point in my Mom's life. For the last ten years she had worked hard at Nationwide to become a success. By the time I turned thirteen, Mom did not struggle as she did when she first started her journey in Ohio. She was in a great job, making good money, and her ties to her past were all but gone. She had done what few are able to do by themselves.

As I started to grow, my dependence on her started to fade. I no longer needed her for many of the things I had in the past, and David was not too far behind. He was nipping at my heels, eager for the opportunity to have more independence. With the two of us starting the inevitable separation, Mom started to see the reason for her hard work start to slip away as well.

The last ten thirteen years of her life had been based around her two children. She worked to better David and I; her own self interests were put on hold, and we were put in its place. She started to see ahead and saw the house empty. She started to see the reality that one day she would not have us around as much; she would be alone.

The fear of loneliness can drive people to do many things they would otherwise never do. It has the same pungency as love just in the reverse. Most people will do anything for love and anything to prevent utter loneliness. With us growing up so fast, Mom knew there was going to be a time when she would be alone.

She had dated some of the men she had met at Nationwide but nothing had ever worked out. She asked me one day if it would be all right if she dated someone. I was about sixteen, and I told her to go for it. I could not remember her ever being married to Dad, so I did not see it as her trying to replace him. I was dating at the time, so I figured she would should also. Plus, if she would date someone, maybe she would not be into everything I did so much.

I was able to ask her later why she never remarried, and she told me she never wanted David and I to feel like Mom had brought someone else into the house without our permission. She did not want another man to ever have any say in what she did with her children. The mere thought of another person yelling at David and I terrified her. She probably figured we had been through enough leaving Lynchburg and starting over in Centerburg. Whatever the reason was, she never remarried or dated anyone for an extended period.

This lack of companionship led her in another direction. Most people when they are lonely or are looking for someone to love, get out and starting dating with the hopes of meeting that special someone. Mom did not do that; she turned to the heavens to fill the void of loneliness.

David and I had been to church a few times before but never to the extent we were about to start. All the two of us knew about God was what we picked up from friends or the vacation bible school Marilyn took us to in the summers. God, the Bible, and anything else to do with Christianity were foreign to my brother and me.

Going to church was something that happened suddenly with Mom. She would tell the story that God had placed a burden on her heart to get her two children into church before they were lost to the world. In reality, she was returning to the God she had left behind when she married Dad. God put the burden on her to come back, and she leapt for her Lord. Her faith would be what would fill the voids of loneliness and give her strength to continue. God would become the reason she got up in the morning, no longer would it be David and I. With the two of us substituted, she had something that would last for the rest of her life. God would not be leaving her like her two sons eventually would.

Religion was not something new to my mother. As a young girl she went to church and had been in church until she starting seeing my Dad. Her mother, Gladys, was a devoted giver to Thomas Road Church, a part of Jerry Falwell ministries. While in Ohio, Mom kept up with the activities of Jerry Falwell and his church and university through her dad and new wife Joanne, both members of Thomas Road. When Mom starting looking for a church, she kept Thomas Road in mind as a model for what she was looking for.

One Saturday afternoon while driving home from Mount Vernon after a trip to the grocery store, she drove by a church and decided that would be the church she would attend the next morning. She did not know anything about the church. She just knew the sign said Southern Fundamental Baptist—exactly what she was looking for. She told David and I we were going to church the next morning to see how things went. We both agreed, but it really was not an option. Even though she asked what we thought about going, we really did not have a say. The next morning we would be getting dressed up and going to church whether we liked it or not.

The next morning as we drove to church, everything I knew about God and religion went through my head. Most of the images were from various horror movies or satires I had seen or read about the Holy Rollers or fanatical extremists determined to bring on the end of the world. I did not understand what Mom was going back to. It was like she was going home after a huge fight, long after the fight was over. David and I were really there that first day just so she would not have to sit in the pew by herself. It makes it easier to confront mistakes when someone else is present. She was returning to her God after she had walked out on Him. She did not know what to expect or even if she would be welcomed back.

After a quick stop at McDonald's for some Egg McMuffins, she hesitantly drove to the church. I could not understand why she was so nervous. She fidgeted in her seat the entire time we were in the parking lot eating our breakfast. One would have thought she was going to be walking in front of a firing squad or that God was going to strike her down the moment she crossed the threshold. When we were done eating, she waited until a few people had walked in before getting out of the relative safety of her car and headed in. I guess she was thinking that if anything bad was going to happen, it would happen to those who walked in first. They would get the lightening bolts from the heavens instead of her.

Just as she stepped in, both David and I at her side, her face changed from that of terror of what lay ahead, to one of total peace. When the preacher offered his hand, she shook it and did her introductions. After a few minutes of small talk we took our seats in the sanctuary and waited for the services to start. We had missed Sunday school, but we had made it in time for the morning service. While we were waiting, many of the church members introduced themselves to us as they took their seats.

On this morning we had the pleasure of meeting Ida for the first time. She made the three of us feel like a part of the group. She even sat with us to make us feel more comfortable. She took the time before the start of the service to fill us in on how things worked. She made sure we knew where to go for Sunday school the next Sunday, and filled us in on who was who and who did what. Ida would become one of the closest friends my mother would ever have, bounded by a common thread to immerge in the near future.

When services finally started, the choir burst into a song that brought my mother to tears. As the words "Praise Him, praise Him our blessed redeemer!" rang through the sanctuary, my mother through sobbing tears apologized to God for running from Him. She made a commitment to Him to never leave the path He had laid out before her again.

She had been running for so long, she had forgotten what it was like to be at home. She ran from her parents when she married Dad. She ran from Lynchburg when her marriage failed, but she was unable to run from God. He felt it was time for her to stop running in the wilderness and return home in His presence. On that Sunday she came home, and her heart was broken with the errors of her past. Finally she was able to make amends with her past and say goodbye to it forever. She gave her mistakes to God and walked out of church a new spirit within the loving fold of her God.

Her life became complete within the span of a few moments in the house of the Lord. The weights on her shoulders and the fear of her future were gone. She put her burdens in the Lords hands and began a journey through life with the rededication to God and His plan for her life and the life of her two children.

The change in Mom was not always clear. She was always a pretty good person around David and I, but there were some distinct differences. The profanity was gone. She drank on very rare occasions but now that was out, and what was acceptable for David and I changed. She now disapproved of all the horror movies and rap music I had. The books I enjoyed so much were now a thing of the past for her. She would no longer buy anything that was not "glorifying the Lord" as she put it. She even went so far as to throw some of my stuff away when I was not paying attention. I would have to look through the trash before I set it out to fish out my movies, CDs, and books.

Emmanuel Baptist Church became my mother's home. William Risley and his family became an extension of her social circle and helped reestablish her faith in the Lord. David and I had school and the friends we had in school. Mom had church and the members of the church. This gave her a place other then work that made her feel at home and gave her a purpose.

Eventually her faith in God would clash with the way I saw the world and my goals for my life. The relationship between mother and son during the teenage years usually centered around school, girls, staying out later, and doing what you are told when you are told to do it. With church now in the mix, our battles would not center on normal teenage issues. They would focus around faith and God. Mom was getting ready to drawl a line in the ground, and I was more than willing to challenge it and even cross it with little regard.

24

The Summer of New Found Dreams

The summer between my seventh and eighth grade year was spent with Dad in Lynchburg. This would be the last summer I would spend with Dad, and his visits to Ohio would be much fewer in number and for shorted amounts of time. David and I were growing up and did not have the time to spend with Dad like we did as children. His visits would be limited to birthdays and major holidays. Our ties with him were broken that summer, and he saw the same things Mom saw earlier that year. Our lives were becoming more independent and time to spend with the parents was rapidly getting less and less.

This summer would also be the summer where I would pick up my life's dream. It would also be the summer my voice would finally start to change. Unfortunately, instead of changing deeper, it decided to go several octaves higher for a couple of years. This Mickey Mouse squeak of a voice would give me problems for several years before it finally decided it had gone the wrong way and go deeper—more like a man's voice.

Even with Mom's rediscovered faith, I still read horror novels and watched the bloodiest movies I could find. Dad was my primary supplier of books and movies, and during the summer I was able to add to my collection. I was able to pick up enough books to last me at least a years worth of terrifying tales. In the course of buying new books, I spent many late nights reading some of the new tales I had picked up. My summer nights were filled with the images of ghouls and demons terrifying small towns or hacking up teenagers too stupid to run away from the danger.

After reading one novel in particular that summer, I told Dad to take it with him to the flea market and sell it. Dad stopped for a minute and asked why I wanted to resell the book. I never sold my books. It was a thing of pride for me to have all the books I had read. I told him the book was awful. It was the worse novel I had ever read. The monsters were weak; the plot was very plain, and it just in general was not too entertaining.

Instead of taking the book to sell, he gave it back to me and told me to do better. Dad said that if I could be such a tough critic then I ought to be able to do better. If I could not do better, then I should not be so hard on someone who was at least trying. With that I had been told to write a story that was better then the one I had just read. This challenge would lead to a desire to be a great American novelist. This dream would be a dream that would make it through my teenage years and into adulthood. In a span of five minutes, I was given something to reach fore for the rest of my life.

With the task of writing a story, I purchased some paper and pens and went to work on a story I called *A Murder Story*. It took me the entire summer to finish and was roughly one-hundred and fifty pages when it was finished and typed out professionally. Computers were not around at the time, and Dad did not want to waste money on a typewriter until he knew I would stick with it. Like so many growing up, I jumped from one idea to another, spending money on items that would be used for a week then discarded to the garage or basement to collect dust. When he saw I had actually filled several notebooks with my story, he had someone type it for me and made several copies.

Dad thought the story was great, but I understood he was looking through biased eyes. When I read it today, I can see my boyish outlook on life ringing through with every word. It was not hard to tell a youth had written the story, but it still had the beginnings of a great horror flick. Everything needed was there. There was a creepy psycho and plenty of blood and gore to go around. I did not become really excited in my work until a local publisher in Columbus decided to print some copies for the local bookstores. I did not get paid much. In fact, I barely covered the cost of a good copyeditor, but at least I had something I had written out for others to buy. It only sold a few copies, but it was enough for me. This story had given me the confidence to seek a career in literature and inspired my wildest dreams. For then on I would put those dreams down on paper with the hopes of entertaining the world.

Later that same year everything would come to a stop when Mom read the story her son had written. She would put my dreams of being a horror writer on hold and purposely put up blocks with the intention of steering me away from the dreams of monsters and death with the goal of intriguing my readers. She did this in the name of her God and this would start strife between the two of us that would last many years and cause many hurtful fights.

With Dad's help that summer, I continued dreaming and put my dreams on my paper. He was similar to me. He always looked at rusted, busted up cars and saw potential and dreamed of what the cars would look like when he finished restoring them. I wrote my stories and imagined what people would say when the read them. I dreamed of the day when I would be able to walk down the isles of the book store and see my novels tucked in the shelves among the other horror writers. With this first story, I was given a taste of something I wanted more than anything. From now on, I would constantly be pursuing that dream and looking forward to the time when I would see it come true.

Dad had given me the ability to day dream. Mom was giving me the determination to see it through and complete what I had started. I even saw the danger of unfulfilled goals through Dad. I saw his yard and house filled with pieces of his dreams never to be realized. I did not want that to happen to me. I wanted to be someone who actually attempted to achieve instead of talking the talking.

That summer with Dad was not only an opportunity to discover my love for the written word, but it was also the last summer for me to be a kid. The summers following this one would be filled with part time work, writing seminars, girlfriends, and church activities arranged by Mom. I no longer would be able to sleep in late and play late into the night. The days of fishing and swimming were soon to be gone. This was my last chance to be a kid. These were the last few months of my childhood.

With Dad not working, drawing his disability, I had the opportunity to do more that summer than at any other time. Several weeks were spent at Virginia Beach, countless hours were spent out at Smith Mountain Lake, and most nights were filled with load music and cook outs. The days started late and lasted long into the night. I did not work that summer other than occasionally doing the dishes or taking a few hours to mow the lawn; the rest of the time was spent writing, doing nothing, or playing as only a child can in the long days of the summer.

I never once had to get dressed up and spent most of the summer in shorts and tees shirts topped off with a baseball cap. By the end of the summer I had completely let go of the things of the past. My toys were not longer G.I. Joes or Star Wars figures or baseball cards; they became stereos, ATVs, and anything to do with the ladies. I was a young adult when I returned to Centerburg to start the eighth grade.

When I left that summer I had some childish tendencies; when I returned I was a young man. All the desires of childhood had run through my system, and it was time to move onto something else. I returned with a new passion. When I had left, I was sure I was going to be an astronaut. I returned with the desire to be a writer, toting my first story under my arm.

An era in my life had ended and new one had started. I could never go back to what I was, and Mom and Dad could not recapture the son they had once enjoyed. I was a new person, slightly closer to the man I would eventually become. The rules of life had changed; they had become more complicated. The gray areas were starting to encroach, and Mom and Dad had to adjust with me. Sometimes I think I was harder for them than it was for me. I was eager to embrace the new, while they struggled to hold onto the past. A life of tug of war started, and it would have some rough times before it would finally be over.

25

Faith Vs A Teenager

The eighth grade started like any other school year. This my second year in high school, and the fears of starting a new year were well behind me. I looked forward to getting back into the routine of school. I had had a huge summer and had something to show my friends. I had a story in print and was eager for my friends to read it and let me know what they thought.

Throughout the summer, Mom had remained faithful to her church attendance. She even came for a visit to Lynchburg during her dad's birthday over the Fourth of July. While she was there she insisted we attend church with her. Together, with our grandparents, we attended Thomas Road Baptist Church in the morning, and then spent the rest of the day at a cook out to celebrate my grandfather's birthday. That was the only time that summer David and I entered a church or really even thought about God. Unlike Mom, Dad did not have much faith or any kind of dedication to God. He did his thing and let God do His thing.

When we returned, getting back in the habit of going to church so much took a little while to get used to. I looked forward to school, but dreaded the hours I would spend each week in a pew keeping my head up while the preacher seemed to drone on forever. Mom tried her best to get me involved with the church activities, hoping it would make it a little more of pleasure instead of something she forced me to do every Sunday and Wednesday night. When her attempts to get me involved in the church failed she turned to my passion. Her heart was in the church, mine was in my books and the stories I was writing.

She had read *A Murder Story* before I started school and was horrified at what she read. The violence and gore upset her, but instead of taking a head on approach to the problem, she decided to show me how what I was writing was not what the Lord would want me to be doing with my talent. Just like her attempts to get me to become an active member of the church, her attempts at changing the topic I wrote about failed. Gentle nudges were not going to be enough to get me to see the horror movies, books, and stories I was writing, were not what a good Christian would engage his time. She would have to use force to make her point, reasoning had failed.

It all started with a simple question. Mom wanted to know exactly where I stood with my beliefs in the Bible. She asked if I believed. Knowing if I said yes, she would not believe me; I would actually be backing myself into a corner, and if I said no, she would go into a long regiment of Bible study until I did believe; I answered her question with another question. It was the safest move for me thinking on the fly. I did not understand that my return question would just lead to more questions and ultimately a debate that would last years between the two of us.

My response was simple. I just asked if she believed in Santa Claus. I knew she did not, but she also knew I had put her in a position that would have to be addressed very carefully. Her response would dictate who won the argument. She had told me for years Santa Claus was real. When I found out other wise, I knew she had lied to me for years. She had given me the hope of a jolly fellow in order to make the holidays a little more magical as a kid, but the lie was eventually discovered. For a moment I had the upper hand.

Instead of answering, she asked if I had any questions about the Bible. She figured maybe if she answered, or got the answers to some of my questions, she would be able to build a case in favor of the Lord. I told her I would think about it for a while and ask while I was in Sunday school. This gave me some time to think about a question that would stump those who were supposed to have complete faith and get me out of the conversation for a few days so I could go back to whatever I had been doing before she interrupted. Mom thought I was asking questions in Sunday school because I thought they were more reputable sources; she did not know I did not have any questions at the time. I really had never thought about it before. I started Sunday service ready for it to be over. Everything was just filler to me.

The next Sunday we all went to church like we always did, but before going in Mom asked if I had anything I wanted to ask and I said I did. I would ask my question in Sunday school that morning. She told me I would be joining her in the adult class this Sunday. The preacher taught the adult class so she was confident I would get a good answer, plus she would be able to hear what I asked. With that, David went to his class and Mom and I took a seat in the adult class and waited to get started—Mom engaging in mindless conversation while I sat in boredom, or politely answered the questions the adult addressed to me.

I was only fourteen at the time, and though I had picked up my creativity and ability to dream from my dad, from her I had picked up a very logical and quick witted mind. For as long as I could remember, Mom had pounded in my head to learn everything I could about a subject, look at it critically, and come up with my own conclusions. She taught me to be careful of information I could not prove and not to have blind faith in what others said or wrote. In giving me this mind set, she had created an opponent to her faith that would stretch her wits and seriously test what she believed.

When class finally began after a brief prayer, the preacher asked if there were any questions. It was obvious Mom had spoken to him before we met. Their eyes were on me waiting for the question I wanted to ask. After a few seconds of silence, I asked if God ever changed his mind. The preacher said no and the others in the class all agreed. The group as a whole even went as far to say, that what was true when the Bible was first written was still true and right today. God never said something was bad then came back and said it was good or the other way around. I thanked him for his answer, and he began the class he had planned. Both he and Mom looked disappointed at the question I asked. They both expected something a little more complicated.

The class went on for several minutes before I spoke up and said I had another question. With a broad smile, the preacher stopped his lesson giving me the go ahead to ask the question. I asked how many people were created when He created the world. I was told Adam was created first, and then later Eve was created from Adam so he would have companionship. When he finished his explanation, I concluded what he said by stating God had created two people, a male and a female. By this time the entire class was into explaining the first two to ever live on the planet. Mom was the only one who was hesitant about my questions. She started to get the sense I was setting them up. She did not know where I was going with my questions, but they knew they had a purpose.

Pastor Risley asked if there was anything else I wanted to know, and I told him I was good at the moment. I would let him know if I needed to know anything else. Mom wanted to get on with the class; she was fairly sure I had another question, and she knew she did not want me to ask. I do not think Mom figured out where I was going with the questioning or she probably would have asked me to step outside a moment before I had the chance to ask. But I could tell by the looks on her face she was worried about what would come out of my mouth next.

Thus far, I had been assured God never changed His mind and that there were only two people created in the beginning. The preacher had agreed with this as did everyone else in the class. They even sighted verses to give me a Biblical reference to answer the simple questions I had. When there was another brief pause in the lesson, I told the pastor I had one last question. Again he smiled and nodded for me to go ahead with the question.

I asked if incest was acceptable to God. The patronizing smile on the preacher's face as he expected another childish question vanished and Mom's foot came slamming down on my toes. I would have to make sure I did not sit next to her the next time I joined her in the adult class. This time everyone in the class was silent. They were not trying to teach the youth among them anymore. Instead, they too were looking towards the pastor for an answer to the question. I had successfully pinned them all of them into a corner. I did this with simple questions that had simple answers but led to a tangle that could not easily be unknotted.

Before I could get an answer to my question, Mom took me out of the class and put me in the sanctuary to wait until morning services to begin. I am sure I had started a conversation in the adult class that morning and would have liked to be apart of the discussion. It would have been enlightening. I later found out they were trying to figure out how to answer the question without opening doors to even more questions, but still maintaining Biblical principles. When the morning service was over, the preacher asked me to come back to his office for the answer to the question I had asked.

He told me incest was not wrong in the eyes of God. Brothers could marry their sisters, but that it was not healthy in today's society. He explained it took many years for the consequences of sin to have it's full effects on man, that is why they lived so long and did not have the birth defects caused by not spreading the genes around like in today's society. He explained incest was alright, but to create a child knowing the child would have defects was against the will of the Lord. It was an answer, but not a real firm one, but it did answer where Cain's wife came from. It had always been obvious to me he had married one of his sisters.

Before we went into next Sunday's services, Mom asked what my question would be before we entered the class. She wanted to be clear about what I was going to ask. Dropping such a bombshell of a question among so many people who were very conservative and not used to such open and controversial questioning would not happen this Sunday morning.

Again my question was simple. I just wanted to know if God was omnipotent and if I had to pray to Him. I would stay away from the questions revolving around sex. In a Baptist church, sex is not talked about openly other than to condemn those who engage in activities in contradiction to the Bible. Prayer and God's ability to know everything from the very beginning of time to the very end of time would be a safe subject. Mom was satisfied, and we went to class and waited to get started.

This time when the other adults joined the class, they were all ready for my questions. They had a pet project now. Instead of just the preacher, everyone was there to help me see the light. I had stumped them with the question during the previous class. During this class, instead of learning a planned lesson, they would all use their skills to answer the questions I would pose to them. Answering my inquiries became the lesson for the class. I was their opportunity to address the issue unbelievers had when they went out soul winning. This was a practice session. If they could adequately cover the issues I was bringing up during the class, they would be prepped for real world evangelism.

After the prayer to start the class, everyone looked at me. They were waiting for me to ask. With a quick prompt from Mom, I asked if God new everything that was going to happen in my life. I asked if He knew every decision I was going to make and every mistake I would make throughout my life. Did He know every second of my life from my birth to my death, and did He know all of this when He first created the world.

After sighting some verses, they all assured me my life was completely mapped out and known to God from the very moment He created the world and all the things of the world. God knew exactly what I would do and the paths I would take throughout my life as He did for everyone else who came before me and that would come after me. God knew every door I would walk through and every opportunity I would pass up. He had the complete map of my life before my parents were even born. He knew it all and saw it all before it ever happened.

With that answer I asked why I should pray to God. Why should I bother Him with my prayers? He already knew what I was going to do; He already knew the roads I would go down. Why waste the time to talk to God if everything was already known way before I was even created. What He knew when He created the world would be true when I was actually born. My decisions were already made for me during creation. I could pray all I wanted, but I would still do what ever God knew I was going to do when He first conceived the world. He knew the out come of my life when He breathed the first breath of life into Adam's lungs. Why did I need to give Him updates through prayer or make requests through prayer? Everything was taken care of before my life started.

The first question was easy for the group to answer. It was obvious to them God knew everything, but when I combined it with the question of prayer it became a paradox without easy explanation. Answering the first question made answering the second far more difficult. It took the rest of the class to get an answer, and the answers were very vague. They were almost like the response that God works in mysterious ways or that it was the Lord's will. The answers did not really answer the question, but simply left more questions.

Ida, our first friend when we joined the church, gave me the best explanation to this very tough question. She put the answer into a reference I could understand. She chose an explanation that did not require a deep understanding of Biblical principals. She explained to me that Mom knew a lot of the barriers and challenges I would come up against through life. Though Mom did not know everything I would be doing, she had already grown up and knew much of what I was going though. Even though the adolescence challenges had to be overcome in order to step fully into adulthood and those challenges could not be changed, it always helped to talk with her when things got really tough. Just by talking to Mom, even if I did not get a concise solution, it often helped just getting it off my chest. Prayer was similar to talking over problems with Mom. It was a way to ease the worries of the world and giving those worries to God. Prayer was a way of receiving the blessed reassurance that everything would be alright and that I was going to make it.

This was the best response I received that day. It even made sense. Praying was like talking to an all knowing, loving father who was eager to hear from His sons and daughters. Prayer was also a way of receiving encouragement to keep pressing forward. Everyone needs encouragement; getting it from the Lord is very reassuring since He already knows the outcome. It is always great to get a pat on the back or an uplifting word from someone who has already been through the problems or had to overcome the challenges you yourself are up against. They know what it is like and know how things will turn out.

A turning point had been crossed that day. I was starting to see how God fit into ones life. It was making sense with every question I had for the preacher and the people in the class. The point of the Bible was one of faith. Yes, it gave life instructions and is a history for some of the greatest men and women doing the Lords work, but it was a book of faith—God's only request. He only asked to be loved and to be accepted over the world around us. The next Sunday, I would see the joy of giving ones life over to God and His son Jesus.

My last question was simple. I just wanted to know why God did not do miracles in today's times. I knew God did major miracles very infrequently within man's history. There is a lot of time covered in the Bible and many of the miracles happened over great periods of time, but there still should have been at least one during the last couple of hundred years. Why had He stopped? Why had He stopped showing His supremacy to his people when they needed it the most?

Soul winning would be a lot easier if we could point to a recent event, even if the event was a couple hundred years old, and say "Look! There is the proof of God and the only true path to His glory." But, for some reason, God had gone quiet.

There were several attempts at trying to explain why God had stopped splitting seas, bringing plagues to oppressors, and stopped speaking from mountain tops to His people and the followers of His son, but none of them seemed to work for me. They all seemed to move around the subject without actually addressing the question. Again, we were back at the Lord's will and that He works in mysterious ways. I had a hard time and still have a hard time believing God does things without giving an answer to those who ask. God promised wisdom and knowledge if we asked. God may wait to give an answer but eventually He does. More than enough time had passed since the miracles of Jesus and God's super miracles for Him to have given His followers an answer.

After some debating about the subject, the class seemed to give up trying to answer the question. The preacher had sited several versus and given an explanation only a well trained Biblical scholar could understand, when Ida spoke up. It was just the previous Sunday when Ida had offered her thoughts. Her explanation made sense to me then, so I gave her my full attention. She went over a concept I had never heard before, and I would be reminded of her explanation much later in my life at a time when I really needed to be reminded.

Ida read books like most people watched television. She had an affection for words I completely understood, but that is lost to most people today. She gave an explanation she had read years earlier that had explained everything to her when she had the same question. She gave me two simple statements and told me to write them down. Ida explained that I would know something is true because I can see that is true. I would believe something was true because God said it was true. These were two simple sentences that when first read did not mean much to me. Seeing I was lost—some of the others looked lost as well—Ida continued her explanation.

She asked what the most basic purpose of the Bible is, and what the most basic want God had of His people while in this world. After a pretty intense debate everyone finally came to an answer. The most basic desire God has is for the people in the world He created to love Him. He has given us the choice as to whether we would love Him or deny Him. He gave the world His son as the only way into the glory of God and has given us the Bible to use as a guild for life and as proof of His Lordship. When we chose to love the Lord, we chose to believe in the Word of God. Our faith, which is also belief, in the sacrifice of Jesus at the cross is the only way to show our love for Him. We must have faith in the promise He has given to all believers through the Word. If this is true, then the choice each of us has to make is whether or not to believe. God wants our complete faith as a symbol of our love for Him.

With the discussion winding down, everyone in agreement, Ida went back to her two sentences she had given me. She asked if I believed she was sitting across from the table from me. Without thinking, I answered yes. She shook her head and asked me to read the first sentence she had given me. After looking at it again, I answered with a no. I did not believe she was across the table, I knew she was across from me because I could see her. She then asked if I knew that the price of Northeastern stock was up three percent at the end of closing on Friday. This time I hesitated before I answered.

After some thought, I answered no; I did not know one way or another. She told me it was and asked if I knew now. She shook her head as I said yes. Ida asked if I knew the stock was up or if I believed what she was telling me. After a few seconds of thought, stuck on the question, she asked if I had seen the Wall Street Journal or some other financial reporting instrument that I could have seen the results of the Northeastern stock. I answered no, and she said then I must believe what she was telling me. I did not know the information was correct, but I believed what she was saying. In a way, you could say I had faith in the information she was giving me.

As a wrap up, Ida explained God had given us the Bible to show our faith. God did not do major miracles, because if he did something like write his name in the sky, people would no longer believe in God; they would know God. God wants belief demonstrated through faith. This is the decision everyone must make in their lifetime. They must either choose to believe or not to believe.

This was a profound concept for not only me but for all the others in the class. Later I would remember the conversation and start to understand the pastor had said the same thing, but Ida simplified the answer in a way everyone could understand and grasp with the use of two sentences.

Ida gave me a clarification that Sunday morning that would lead me into taking my first step of faith in the Word of God and the gift of Salvation. She gave me a solution to the basics of Biblical understanding that fit my logical, analytical mind. Though my mother had tried through force and by immersing me in and around the people and the works of the church, Ida's two sentences led to my faith in Jesus.

That Sunday afternoon I made the decision to look to the Lord for His saving grace and started a new life as a believer. From now on, the Bible would be considered fact to me. The parts I could not easily explain would be a step of faith on my part that they were true, just as God had said they would be.

26

Expectations Run High

With my new found faith in Jesus, Mom expected lots of things to change in my life. She expected me to be more attentive in church and to be more social with the people of the church. This was not something I was going to do easily. I was more attentive when the preacher spoke, wanting to learn more about the faith I had, but I did not want to be associated with the people of the church other than the occasional dinner or church picnic. They just were not my type of crowd.

My desire to write continued, and horror remained the primary subject. Life was pretty much the same. I wanted to learn more about the Bible and its people, but my daily life and the activities of my daily life did not change much. Life went on as it always did, and this was not good enough for Mom. She wanted more out of me. She wanted me to do the things for God she had not done. She wanted me to be something I was never going to be and do things I was not interested nor inclined to do. After I made the decision to be a follower, she thought everything in my life would change, and I would follow her lead in serving the Lord, but it did not work that way. I was going my own ways and not following the lead she was so desperately trying to give.

Her frustrations came out when she read one of my works in the making and reread *A Murder Story*. She did not want a horror writer in her family; it was contrary to her beliefs and not the path she wanted me to take. After she read some of my new work and my old work, she made a decision to clear the house of the things she felt were not of God and were hurting my spiritual life. With a force and conviction only a Baptist mother can have, she gathered all of my books, magazines, videos, copies of *A Murder Story*, all of my short stories, and even the *Awaking*—a three-hundred page story that was to be my first full novel, and burned everything in the back yard.

Everything I had collected over the years to build my horror collection and help inspire my stories was burnt in a pile reminiscence of Hitler and his book burning ceremonies. She told me this was for my own good and things that were contrary to God and His plan for my life had to been destroyed in order to move in a positive direction in doing the Lord's work. It took several hours for the pile to burn out, leaving only a few melted tapes and small pieces of charred books and magazines.

Though the fire took my inspiration and guilds to the horror writer's craft, as I watched the flames flicker to smoldering smoke, my resolve only got stronger. My mother was a very smart woman, but for some reason she had forgotten copies of *A Murder Story* could be reprinted. She also over looked the typewriter my dad had bought me for my fourteenth birthday. It was not a computer in the sense we know computers today, but it did store everything on disk as a backup. I would type my stories up; edit them on paper, then reprint the edited copy. That night she burnt the works of many great horror writers, but she had not destroyed mine.

That night after she had fallen asleep I reprinted *Awakening* and put in my backpack to take to school the next day. I would have to hide everything I wrote from her in a locker on the first floor of Centerburg High School. I discovered that night my prize possessions were no longer things, but they were my creative words on paper to make a story. The things I loved were characters I had made up and story lines I had crafted during many late nights. I had to protect these things from a faith driven mother bent on moving her son into a life she herself had given up years before my birth. I thought my locker would be the safest place to hide that most precious to me.

When I woke up the next morning, I thought the "cleansing" had been completed. I figured everything was over; I would just have to explore my ideas and dreams outside of the house. This would not be too hard. I could name many of my friends who were different people when they were around the influences of their parents and completely opposite when their parents had their backs to them. I would simply live a life at school that supported the dreams of being a writer, and fill the vicarious living conditions of a Bible beating son while at home to pacify Mom.

With expectation of having a normal day at school and starting a new plan to be able to continue my creative outlet, I went to school with a backpack loaded with stories. Before classes started, I put the stories at the bottom of my locker and placed my books over them to protect them from getting torn or bent as stuff was thrown in and taken out during the day.

I used my time in study hall to continue my stories and placed the updated copies back in my locker each afternoon. Even though they had to be written completely freehand, they still came together well, and I was able to add greatly to them just using a pen and notebook paper. I would eventually take them home and type them up when they were completed.

I though I had everything worked out, until I was told to come to the office instead of getting on the bus to go home. The note to stay came just before the last period was over, completely preventing me from getting anything from the class. During lunches a couple of my friends and I would sneak off school grounds and get something to eat at the Kent's Cones just down the street or go to the store and pick up donuts. We had to be careful when we did this; getting caught meant a good deal of time would be spent in detention. With this note, it looked like we had been caught; someone had seen us sneaking off or saw us while we were out.

After the class ended, I took my time to my locker and put my books away, grabbed my coat, and took the long way to the principal's office. This was the first time I had been in any trouble other than talking in class or not doing my homework on time. I had only been to the office to give excuse notes when I was late or sick from school. I had never had to go there and talk to anyone. After several minutes of killing time, I made it to the office, looking for my friends who had been out to lunch with me, figuring they would all be there as well, but did not see them.

I walked in to see my mother in the principal's office with several of my teachers. From the way it looked, she had been there for a while and they were all caught up in their conversations. They did not notice I had finally arrived after avoiding showing up for as long as I could. Mary, the office secretary, interrupted them and led me into the office. Mom was being more thorough then I had thought. She had had the same idea I had had. If I could not follow the dream of horror and science fiction writing at home, then school would be the next best place. This meeting was to prevent the encouragement I would have at school. This was her plea to my teachers not to encourage works that included violence or things that would be contrary to her beliefs.

She had her talk with my educators, and they were instructed to let her know if I engaged in writing that was of the horror nature. She wanted to be informed of everything I did that was evidence I was still writing about ghouls and goblins. She had intruded into the one place I thought I would have refuge from a faith driven mother with the intention of forcing her views onto her son at whatever the cost.

On the way home that evening, she told me the things of the past were now truly things of the past. No one would be able to read the stories I had written, and she would deny anything I had done to contribute to the horror genre. The short story *A Murder Story*, to her never existed, was never published, and would never been seen again. *Awakening* would never have a chance to be published or read. In her mind, she had purged her son of the evils of the words he was writing.

I sat in the car, vowing not to give into her ways. She had pushed too hard. The harder she tried to prevent me from following my dreams, the more determined I became. No longer did the horror movies, magazines, and books become my inspiration, Mom did. She became the primary reason I kept going and pushing forward with the dream of being a writer. I was determined to prove her wrong. I would become a published author one day, and people will read the stories I have created, and there is nothing she can do about it. She may slow me down, but she would not stop me.

It did not take long for Dad to get wind of what Mom was doing. He was my biggest encourager and did what he could to help further develop my skills. He had been the reason *A Murder Story* had been published. He was also the primary way I had of getting movies to watch and books to read. The books Mom had destroyed had been purchased and given to me by him. She told Dad she had done it in the name of God, and that he should show a little more concern about the things his son read and watched. She used this against him, causing many long fights about what had happened. He saw what I was doing as a good thing; she saw it as an evil thing. The two would be pitted against each other for quite some time.

I still was able to write during study halls and keep my works in the bottom of my locker as I added to them each day. During the summer before I started my freshman year in high school, I kept my work in the back of my closest and added to them while Mom was at work. That summer also gave me opportunity to start typing out my stories and editing them. By the time my freshman year started *Awakening* was completed. I made sure to save everything on disk and hide the disks just in case Mom got wise and found the stories and tried to erase them from my typewriter.

During the summer, things seemed to calm down a bit. Dad came up for a couple of visits and took me to see the latest horror or science fiction flick while Mom worked. I spent many days at the Centerburg Library reading the books Mom would not let in the house. To her everything had gone as she had planned. No longer were there any movies or books in her house that went against her beliefs. I was going to church as she had wanted.

The illusion of success on my mother's part was working until I had completed an English assignment my freshman year. I was given an assignment to write about a process. Mrs. Huddleston was my English teacher for the second time. I thought I had seen the last of her red pens after I finished the seventh grade, but fate would have it, she also taught freshman English. I only had to write three pages and I dove into the assignment with excitement.

During the summer, I had been able to get away with writing my stories. I was beginning to get cocky with my ability to do what I wanted without Mom knowing, but I was eventually going to make a mistake that would bring everything tumbling down. I messed up when I used this assignment to rewrite a small piece of *Awakening*. In *Awakening*, one of the main characters was in the process of become a warlock. I used this paper to write a general outline of what one would have to do to become a warlock. This was the paper I turned in for the process assignment.

When the paper was returned to me the next day, I was surprised to see it had very few red marks and had a huge A written across the top. Getting a paper back from Mrs. Huddleston without red ink everywhere meant I was perfecting my craft. The many hours spent during the summer writing was beginning to pay off. I was beginning to develop my own style and the skills needed to write professionally. I did not know the paper had been copied and given to the guidance counselor and principal before given back to me with its grade.

The next day before my last period ended, I received a note to stop by the office before going home. Just like before, I thought the gig was up. Someone had seen my friends and I out during lunch. Unlike before, I was not nervous about going to the office. I now knew the people who worked in the office, and detention was no longer something I dreaded. I had never been to detention, but I would not mind hanging out in the office for an hour or two after school. The mystery of the people and what they could do no longer had a hold over me.

When class was out, I went straight to the office. I would go to my locker after I stopped by to see what they wanted. I did not want to have to sit in detention with a coat and full book bag at my side. I was shocked when I walked through the door and saw my Mom sitting in the office with Mr. Nauman, the principal, and Mr. McDavid, the guidance counselor. Again they were deep into their conversations and did not know I had arrived. Mary motioned for me to go on back, and I hesitantly went into the principal's office—the conversation stopping immediately as they waited for me to take a seat.

I did not realize they brought in the parents when their kids went to lunch off school grounds. I figured a note home with an explanation as to why their kid had to stay after school would be the extent. If they had pulled Mom from work, I would not be in trouble for ditching lunch, but for her having to come to the school to talk about me ditching class. Mom was a very busy woman at Nation-wide by this time. She did not have time to be called to school because I went to the store for lunch instead of eating in the cafeteria. I was now thinking they took leaving school grounds to be a lot more serious then I had thought.

I was floored when Mr. McDavid pulled out the paper I had turned in during English class. Again I was back in the same place I had been a year earlier. Mom had the English teachers turn in anything that she did not approve. The school then contacted her about the incident. As the meeting went on, both the princi-pal and guidance counselor said it was very well written. It was of professionally quality. Mom was the one who jumped in to let everyone know this was not something that was acceptable. It may have been well written, but the subject was forbidden.

The meeting brought a close to the safe haven of school. I would no longer be able to develop my skills within the walls of Centerburg High School. I would no longer be able to write about the subjects I wanted to write about while I was in school. It would not be until my junior year that I would again be able to be my own individual in school through the guidance of Mrs. Reilly, an English and theater teacher. Until my eventual contact with her, I would take on the persona my mom wanted. I would also not write a single paper that was my own work. If the teachers did not want to hear what I had to say or did not want me to express myself the way I wanted, they would not be allowed to read another word that was my own. Until the eleventh grade, everything I wrote was either copied from another person or done just enough to get by. For two years, not one word I wrote was my own idea or thought about any subject assigned to me.

Though I was extremely upset about the meeting, Mr. Nauman and Mr. McDavid knew they were looking at a talent. My mother was blind to the fact I could write and express myself in a way others enjoyed reading. They may have even found my paper entertaining—though they would never let Mom know. They would have to support her in every way possible, but they also saw a gift that was being squashed by a mother who had other plans for her son's future. Recognizing the gift, they saw the potential of what I was able to do. They did not end the meeting like the last meeting a year before.

I am not sure if they understood I was at my wits end with Mom and her pres-sures to be something I did not want, but before the meeting was over, they gave me another outlet that would nurture the gift I had been given. They offered a mentoring program that would pair me up with a professor at Kenyon College who was a published author in the science fiction genre. I would be able to start working with her starting my sophomore year. Though the mentoring program was a school program, it was done outside school during after school hours and was really between just the mentor and the student. This would mean the teachers of Centerburg High would not be able to turn over my work to Mom. It would be between my mentor and me.

I gladly took the offer and left the meeting with Mom. I left with an upset soul but with an opportunity that would expand what I knew how to do much further than anything I could have done within the walls of the high school. I would take a year for me to see, this meeting was a turning point. I am now able to trace most of my creative and expressionistic abilities to the mentoring program that came out of that meeting. I would like to think Mr. McDavid and Mr. Nauman saw what was happening and tried to make a difference in my life while also appeasing my mother. If that is not the case, then it was fate that I would be given the opportunity and later become the writer I dreamed about for so many years.

With the last handshakes given, Mom finally left the office and we went home. For a year she had thought she had a grip on the direction for my life. She so desperately wanted me to become a preacher of the faith; she even thought I was on that path before she received the call from the school. Her expectations for my life had been shattered. She saw the determination I had to ride down my own path through life and with that determination she was loosing her dream of ever seeing her son become a pastor for the Lord.

It would take the entire school year for her to realize what she wanted for me was not what I wanted. I did not see happiness in the future she wanted for me; I wanted no part of it. That freshman year Mom began seeing I was a person with my own ideas, my own dreams, and future that I would make for myself. She was no longer the director for the path of my life. She was slowly taking the backseat only to be able to offer her guidance in times of need, but I would have to make the decisions. She would have to let go, or I would eventually pull away with force.

Later that same month I received another note requesting my presence in the office. I thought they were going to take away the offer they had made during the meeting with my mother. I expected to see her sitting in the office as I walked in, but instead saw my friends. Someone had seen us at the store getting donuts during lunch. We had finally been caught, and I spent my time in detention.

27

Coming of Age

Life during my freshman year was filled with many fights with Mom and our house had the smell of tension. Smiles were rare things when it came to Mom and I. She did not like the turn I had taken, and I moped around the house on edge because of the loss of my stuff and my ability to do what I loved. Words had been my escape from the confusing world of my teenage years, and that had been taken away from me. I did not play sports and had no outlets for my frustrations. It was not until the summer that all of this changed; life started to look a little better.

I am not sure when it happened, but Mom and I started talking. We started talking as friends and not as parent and son. Since we lived out in the country, I was stuck in a house all day with little to do and just David to talk with and my friends could not drive yet.

When she would come home in the evenings from a long day at work, she would catch me sitting on the couch staring blankly at the television or mowing the grass looking like I just got in from a funeral of a dear friend. Like any good mother, she did not like seeing her son so unhappy. After all, everything she had done over the last fifteen years had been to build a life for David and I that was filled with happiness, and here I was with a long face and in a rut.

What my mother was thinking at the time, I am not sure. I just know she was tired of fighting all the time. We were fighting over something she wanted and I didn't. I was not a bad teenager. I did well in school, kept the house in order since she was at work for long days, made sure the lawn was kept up, and made sure David stayed out of trouble. I could have been a lot worse. She had heard horror stories from her co-workers. I was not like that. She decided to bend a little on her plans for the future she wanted for me in the church. She was the one who stopped the fighting.

She broke the ice by talking up the mentoring program I would be a part of starting the next school year. She started to show an interest in what I dreamed of doing. Instead of using force to change the paths I would choose in life, she started to guild. She gave me the ropes but was close by just in case I got into trouble. She opened the lines of communication. Talking would be the way the two of us would come back together, and she started the conversation.

The fights stopped almost immediately, and the smiles started to return. It took the entire summer for peace to come back into our home, but it eventually did and it was embraced with great enthusiasm. We became friends that summer who talked about the issues in my life, and she shared the issues in her life with me. She broke down some of the walls of protection she had built up to prevent David and I from worrying about life's many problems. The blinders that blurred the real world started to open.

She told me many stories about what my younger life was like and many problems she over came that I was not even aware, let alone worried about. I never knew she did not have money to buy food when she was living in the hotel with her two children and was giving blood, rolling change, and barrowing money to make ends meet while she worked hard to get us out of the hotel as soon as possible. I did not realize she went without lunch for years while David and I were in grade school. She used her money to make sure we had lunch money and something to eat for dinner each night.

The many times the power had went out when we were younger was not because of wind and bad weather like she had told David and I, it was because she was not able to make the payment on time. Many of the people who came knocking on our door in times past were not salesmen but debt collectors trying to collect on my mother's debts. The phone calls late at night threatening her because of someone she had fired at work or a customer who was not happy with Nationwide were always attributed to the wrong number. She told us she unplugged the phone at night so people calling the wrong number would not bother her while she slept.

David and I never knew the strains or stresses she was under as she tried to make it in the world with two children. Everyday was a good day for David and I. She always smiled and talked to us as if nothing bad was happening. It is because of her strength as a woman and a dedicated mother, that I have nothing but happy memories of childhood. If she had let the problems of the world seep into the fantasy world she had created for David and I, I am sure those memories would have been filled with nightmares of threatening calls, bill collectors, and possible hunger. She took on the entire weight of the world, and she did it to ensure her two boys grew up in a household filled with memories of good times and bliss.

As we starting talking friend to friend, the problems of the past were in the past. She was making great money at Nationwide and the weights were somewhat lifted from her shoulders. She had become a success against the odds, and she had been able to get through the tough years with no harm to her two sons. We were completely oblivious to the potential worries of the past. I can only hope to be as strong as she was when I have my children and we navigate through life and all of its problems.

As we continued to talk, fights of the past year started to fade. I was finally able to get a mother who listened to what I wanted—she did not give me everything I wanted, but at least she listened and gave an honest response instead of an I said so answer. She gained the closeness of a son, and a friend who she could talk to confidentially. She did not load me up with all her problems, but she did talk things over with me regardless of whether I could help her out or not. I became an ear that was needed in her life. I was someone she could talk to and get things off her chest.

These conversations would begin to prepare me for the life still ahead of me. They also gave me a deeper respect for what she had done to make things work for her family. I also realized I was not the only one who gave up things in life. The things I had let go of in order to move forward were nothing compared to what she released without regret to simply see smiles on the faces of her two boys. My sacrifices in life seemed great to me, but they were nothing in comparison to what my mother had done. Seeing this changed my outlook on life, and I understood what she was trying to do when she took away something she felt was a bad influence. She had worked too hard to create a life for us to let me through it out the window on some silly fantasy.

Just as I started to see her motives for the first time, she started to see I was honestly trying to do something that would make me happy in life. For the first time, she told me I had a gift of creativity and the ability to tell stories people wanted to read. To hear her say I could do something well, even though she did not approve of the content, was enough for me to keep pressing forward while respecting the beliefs she had. We started to come to an understanding. I could pursue literature as long as I kept the swear language to a minimum and tried to keep the gore down as much as possible. I also had to continue to go to church. We met each other half way and the compromise on both parts renewed the happiness in our lives and brought us closer together, something that would be vital in the years to come.

I was not becoming a mama's boy; she still made the rules, and I still did many things she did not think were right. But from now on our fights would last just a day or so and then things would equal out and all would be good in our household. This would be the way life would be while I made it through my teen years. David's experience would be different, but he would make it just as well as I did, even though many of us had our doubts at times.

With an understanding between the two of us, Mom started to support my dreams of being a writer. She knew I would need a way to Kenyon College after school in order to meet with my mentor. She would be at work and needed a way of getting me there each day. Her desire now to encourage what I did and to provide for me the things she had never had as a child inspired her to buy me a car.

It was something that happened without much planning. We were driving home from Mount Vernon after some shopping and she commented on how nice it would be when I could drive and she would not have to cart me all over the place. With a car in mind, I told her a second car would be the answer to the chauffeur service she was providing for David and I. It would also give me a way to get back and forth from Kenyon each day after school. I guess she saw the logic in this or was just looking for the moment when she could buy her son his first car because she pulled into the dealership, and we began looking around at cars. My birthday was still a couple months away, but I was just glad she had brought up the subject and was willing to look. I would not have to hint for my own car; she was already in the mindset of looking. I just had to convince her buy now.

As we strolled through the rows of cars, I was attracted to the new Camaro and with a single look she let me know it was out of the question. As we continued to browse, the salesman came out to lend his assistance. Mom, putting on her best business face, took his business card and told him she was not to be bothered while she looked. If she needed his help, she would be sure to seek him out. With that, the man walked back into the dealership, watching us through the large glass windows as we continued to browse.

As we walked, she started to bargain with me. She wanted to know what I wanted, and she let me know what she was willing to do. I did not have to beg once; it was clear she was going to get me a car. Maybe not today, but she definitely would be getting me one for my birthday. This had turned out to be easier than I had expected.

While we looked, I told her I wanted red. She told me no convertibles. I wanted a CD player. She told me only an automatic; she did not know how to drive a stick and with living with Dad she new the racing and revving potential of a stick. It was this point in the conversation we came across the new Geo Storm. The car was red, automatic, had a CD player, was only a four cylinder, and when she looked at the price it was within what she wanted to spend. She never discussed a price with me, but I knew she had a price in mind. The car was sporty looking but without the power under the hood that would lead to potential reckless driving.

All I said was, "I like this. It looks pretty cool."

With that she went into the dealership, found the salesman, and bought the car. It was that easy. No pleading or debates. I just told her I liked it and wanted it, and she bought it.

Since my birthday was not for a few more months, she arranged the car to be put into storage so I could be the first one to drive it. She did not want to bring it home and start using it before I was able to break it in. For two months, I waited in boyish excitement and counted the days until I would turn sixteen. This car was a symbol of my potential freedom, and I could not wait to get in it and drive. This would be my ticket to the outside world.

Mom did all of this with the expectation the coming year would be a year of diving into my dreams of being a writer and doing well with my new mentor. She also did this to relieve some of the obligations she had on a daily basis. I would soon become her errand boy, but that would be fine with me. At least I would be able get out when I needed. This car also represented an obligation to her. I was now expected to do well in school and to do well at Kenyon. She was putting the ball in my court. If I wanted to keep the car, I would have to pay for it. I did not have to pay in money, but I would have to pay for it in grades, achievements, and the responsibility that came along with the freedom of driving. I would be the one that would decide whether or not I would be able to keep my freedom.

Finally, when early fall finally came around, I was able to start my drivers education a month before my birthday. A friend I had known since grade school was also doing his drivers education at the same time. Even though Pat and I had known each other for quite a while, we had really just started hanging out during the last part of my freshman year and little bits during the summer. While in drivers education we became close friends and built a friendship that would last several years, and he is still considered my best friend from high school. His mother took us to the AAA office in Mount Vernon for the class and picked us up when it was over.

Pat ended up getting is license in September of that year and from then on it was the last time I would ride a bus to and from school. His parents gave him a pickup truck, and he would pick me up every day before school and bring me home after. He did this until my birthday when I would finally be able to drive. Finally one of my friends had a license and was not stuck at home or dependant on rides from parents. With just the little bit of freedom Pat gave me when he received his license, I was became so anxious and looked forward to the day when I would have complete freedom with my own license to drive.

I was up at six AM waiting for the dealership to open on my birthday. I was dressed and ready to go a good two hours before the doors would open. Dad had come up to celebrate his son's first car, and the three of us went out to breakfast. I only had my learners permit, and Dad would have to drive Mom's car back while the two of us took my new car with me behind the wheel.

The salesman who sold us the car put it in storage in a building behind the dealership until I was able to pick it up. Since we finished breakfast a half hour before the dealer would be open, Dad and I were looking through the windows of the garage to have a look at the car I would soon take off in. He had not seen it before, and he seemed just as excited as I was about the new vehicle.

The salesman finally arrived and caught us looking through the windows at the car. He took the time before he opened the main office to open the garage and give me the keys to pull the car out. There was still a little more paper work Mom had to complete before we could leave, but at least I could sit behind the wheel and show Dad my new ride. It wasn't long before a license plate was bolted on the front and back and an offer was made to wash the car before I left. I declined the free wash, told them I would take care of it myself, and told Mom to get in. I was ready. I had been thinking about this day for a couple of months and just wanted to get on the road.

With a final hand shake, we left. I was driving my new car home for the first time, Dad following closely behind in Mom's car. Life was now more then it had been just a few months before. I not only had a way of getting myself around and some greater freedoms into the world, but I also saw the world differently. I had my first long-term, dating girlfriend, I had my license to drive, and I started to see my parents as people and friends that would always be there. I was beginning to see the insignificance of my superficial life of the past. I was getting my first glimpses of the reality both Mom and Dad had protected me from in order to protect my innocence for as long as possible.

This was a coming of age when paths in my life were starting to take shape, and the roads I would take for the rest of my life were just beyond the horizon. Mom and Dad were regretfully letting go of their oldest son and watching him walk through the door of their control into the passage of life. The future was still a blur—there were still many opportunities and many paths to take, but for once I was walking alone; the two of them left behind yelling words of wisdom, but no longer holding my hand. They would not be able to pull me out of harms way anymore. I would either have to avoid it, or suffer whatever consequences may arise from poor decisions. Their job of protectors had now been replaced with the task of being supportive.

28

Dad Would Not Let Go

Mom had started to let go. She was watching me grow up, and by living together, we butted heads every so often in order to move forward to adulthood. Dad had a hard time letting go. Just like I was beginning to see the reality of Mom and recognized her as a person, I was also starting to see Dad for the man he was. I was not a child anymore, and I did not look at him through a child's eyes.

Throughout my early childhood, Dad was a man who came up every month to visit. I always knew him as my father and looked up to him with great admiration, but as time went on, I started to see him for what he was. The things of the past that kept the bond between the two of us together had begun to fade with time. With him not being around as much, he had not learned how to relate to the sons who had grown up in monthly leaps throughout the years.

As a kid, Dad was the fun one to be with. I looked forward to his visits and the summers I would spend at his place in Lynchburg. With him, I was able to stay up late, watch whatever I wanted on television, and do what ever I wanted to do. He had a passion for the same things I had growing up. At times it was hard to tell whether Dad liked Star Wars more than me. His place was filled with the spaceships and action figures that went with the movies.

Ever since I could remember, he had never had a job; he spent all his time when I was with him with me. He would watch the morning cartoons with me, knowing all my favorites and all the characters as well as I did. He was the Dad every son dreams of having, but that would lead to a nightmare when my teen years came.

I was growing up; I was putting the things of the past away and seeking new things, but Dad was still holding on. He was locked in the memories of the past and was constantly trying to recreate the past times. What had once been fun in the past was no longer amusing to me. As a kid I liked staying up late and watching television or catching a midnight showing at the movies, but at sixteen, I had to go to bed at a reasonable time so I could get up the next morning.

When he would visit during the holidays, he would sleep all day and expect me to run around town with him all night long. When I told him I couldn't do this anymore, he would take offence. He would tell me he came to Ohio to visit with David and I, and now that he was here, we would not do anything with him. I tried everything to explain to him that really late nights were a thing of the past for him and I. I had to be at school in the morning; I couldn't be out all night. But for some reason, he never understood. He was living in a vacuum and would not see the reality of the life I had in Ohio.

When he would show up for Christmas or Thanksgiving, I was always glad to see him. I loved him as much as I did Mom, but I was not the same person he watched over during the summers of my youth. I was now doing things on my own without the company of mom and dad. He honestly could not figure out why I would not take him out when my girlfriend and I went out. I tried telling him, taking my dad with me on my dates would not happen. I would gladly take him out to dinner one night during his visits, but he could not monopolize all my time during his stay. I had commitments; I had dates; I had things to do that did not include him.

Mom had been used to me spending less and less time with her. She did what she could to explain to my dad that I was growing up and needed space. She let him know, they were no longer the center of my universe. Everything I did no longer revolved around them. They were once a part of every activity I participated in. Now they were lucky to get a couple of dinners at home each week. This was life. Dad would either have to accept it and move with the flow or be forced into changing.

Dad didn't see the need to change. He felt the child he knew ten years ago was the same one he was coming to visit. He chose to hold onto the fantasies of the past and would not see the reality of the present.

Unlike Mom, there were no talking things over with Dad. There were no compromises between the two of us. He wanted all or nothing, and I could no longer give him that. He felt he had the right to go everywhere I went, when I went, regardless of the situation. He also felt he came before anything else in my life while he was here for his visits, and he started to make his point very clear. Like Mom had years ago, he drew a line in the sand and told me this was the way it was going be.

After trying to talk things over, trying to come up with something that would benefit the both of us, I asked Dad not to come back for a while. I had too many things to do and could not give him the time and devotion he demanded of me. If dinner and the occasional movie or trip to the mall was not enough for him while I was in school, then he should not come back until I had more time to fit him in. We had had great times in the past, but it was in the past. He would not let go, and I could not wait for him to come back to reality.

With my request for him to leave and not to come back for a while, I knew I hurt him. It hurt me. I had to tell my dad to get lost. He was not a bad father, and I had many good times with him, but if he would not grow along with me, he would have to leave. I could not become trapped in the same delusions of past good times. I had to look forward and to move forward with my life.

He had once been my best friend and greatest ally when it came to my writing and the dreams I had of becoming a writer. I will never forget the support he gave when Mom and those at school seemed to be against the very thing I wanted most in life. He was always in my corner, but Mom had come around a bit, and those at school were no longer paying attention to what I was writing; so I was free to explore many stories during study hall and the time with my mentor. I did not need him like I did before. His insistence was becoming a problem. He was starting to get in the way.

Dad was extremely supportive and loved David and I very much, but he had many problems—problems I was not able to deal with as a teenager. I never saw the flaws in him when I was a little boy and looking up at him, but standing eye to eye with him now, I saw what Mom was running from when she left him. He was a man filled with dreams he would never pursue or ever see come true. He had been broken by the weight of life and war and he tried to compensate by talk and no action. I did not want to be that way. I wanted what I said to be supported by the works in my life, and he was not someone who encouraged achievement. He dreamed but never did what it took to become successful.

Looking at him, I could see the hurt he caused Mom. Mom and I had many differences, but when we worked them out and honestly tried to make things better. When I looked at him, I saw a man who had hurt her and never tried to make amends for what he had done. Instead, he seemed to flaunt it before her, blaming her for the many failures in his own life. His problems were never of his own doing; someone else was always responsible. He portrayed the victim to anyone who would listen and buy into his story, but with me it was falling apart. His story was no longer having an effect on me.

Dad would blame Mom for turning his children against him while he was living in Virginia. He would blame her for my actions towards him. He never could see it was not Mom that was turning me against him; I was just not buying into his pity stories anymore. He stood before me as he really was, and I could see through the fog to the soul of the man that was my dad. I will always love him, but I would no longer accept the man he pretended to be.

With this, he left for Lynchburg and did not come back for a good while. I eventually invited him back, letting him know everything was alright between the two of us, but that it would just be different. When I asked him to come back, I told him I was in a play with Mount Vernon Players and had tickets for him and Mom to come up and watch. It was a dinner theater production and told him to bring nice clothes as the occasion warranted. This would be the first time Mom had done anything with me that involved theater or the things I had written. I was looking forward to seeing the two of them together at something I had worked to put together.

When he showed up late Thursday evening, he came into the house with a beard to his chest, tangled and filled with food particles. His hair was matted and unkempt. I initially over looked his appearance and gave him a hug and made sure he had the blankets and pillows he would need for the night. When I got up the next morning for school, I woke him up and asked that he please go get his hair cut and beard trimmed before I got home. Mom had seen him before she left for work and thought the same thing, but I was the one who told him to do it. I took the responsibility to let him know he looked like a bum and needed to get cleaned up before I got home.

On my way to school, Mom called me on the car phone and told me she would be leaving work early to go by Lazarus to pick up some clothes for Dad. She had seen him before she left and figured if he rolled up looking like he had crawled out of a sewer, then he probably didn't bring any nice cloths. She tried to be encouraging. She knew I invited him up in an effort to make things right between the two of us. She did not like the theater or many of my creative works, but she knew they were important to me and this play was a big deal for me. She assured me she would get home early and get him in order before dinner started at the theater.

After school let out, I went home to find the two of them fighting—Dad still looking like he just came from a box under a bridge, Mom insisting that he clean up. When I walked in the shouting stopped, and they looked for me to take sides. I just went to my room, got my stuff and left. I told Dad not to bother coming to the show. If he did not respect me enough to make an effort, then I did not want him there. I did not want to have to explain to my friends why my dad chose to look the way he did. There was no reason for his appearance. He had money; he just chose to be that way.

Later that night, Dad would try to get David to go out with him to run the roads late at night like he always did, and David told him no. Dad had not just lost the companionship of one son but both. Neither of us wanted to be associated with him in the state he was in. We were not asking for Armani suits and manicured nails; we just wanted him to be presentable. If he could not respect himself enough to keep himself up, then he could have done it for the two of us, but he wouldn't.

That night after the play, I called home and told Mom I was going to stay with a friend for the night and to tell Dad goodbye for me. Neither of them were able to make it that night. I gave the table I had reserved for them that night to my girlfriend and her family. I told Mom I would see her Saturday afternoon and finished what was the biggest night of my life with my friends at an after show party.

When I finally rolled in, Mom and Dad were still fighting. Dad insisting Mom had turned his two sons against him because neither of us would have anything to do with him while he was there. I came in to settle the fight. I had thought about what I would say to him all night and here was my chance. This was not the first time he had done something like this in order to cause tension within the house. This was just the last one I was going to take from him. It was time for me to speak up and let him know where things stood.

I asked him if he really thought he would be going out with us looking the way he looked. He said I was ashamed of him, and that I should accept him no matter what. I understood what he was saying, but I also let him know he could do better, and his lack of effort was a reflection of how he really felt about David and I. If this was the best he could, then I would accept him as is, but he was making a mockery of me. He did this to get a sympathy tear from me, but he would not get it from me.

I loaded his stuff back in his truck and asked him to leave my house. He was welcome at anytime; he just had to show David, my mother, and myself the respect we deserved. He was my dad, and I loved him for it, but he would have to start to return the feelings before he would be welcome back. Without much else said, he got in his truck and left. This was the second time I asked him to leave. I had been the bigger man by inviting him back to make amends, but I would not do it again. I had drawn my line in the sand and would not budge, just as he hadn't months before.

I would have thought Dad and I would have had a better relationship then Mom and I. We were much closer when I was younger, and he supported me in everything I did, but it turned out Mom was much more understanding and a far better person to have at my side then Dad. Dad had once supported and encouraged me, but I sought Mom's guidance. She was far more helpful then Dad would ever be.

Ironically, Mom would be the one who would invite him back a couple years later. She would be the one who would try to put things back together. For me, I had rid myself of a man who said he cared but wanted everything his way or no way. I had broken the bonds with Dad by asking him to leave. I had not wanted him out of my life, but he could not be in it if he was going to be destructive.

29

My Mentor Joan

Through the last meeting my mother had at school with my teachers regarding the work I was writing, I was given the opportunity to have a mentor work with me in developing my craft of creative writing. The privilege was mine to be able to work with Joan Sloanzewski, a Micro-Biology professor for Kenyon College. She would be the spark that would keep my pursuits alive. Through her guidance, I would finish the story *Awakening* and even begin another, with the dreams of making it as a published writer.

Joan had successfully been published several times before we ever met. Her genre of choice was science fiction, and she used her vast knowledge of the sciences to further her stories and draw the reader into a world of a far off future or a distant planet filled with diverse cultures. Before I met her for the first time, I bought copies of everything she had had published and read them with the realization I would someday be able to go into a bookstore and pull my books from the shelves in the horror section. I read them several times over as I waited for the day when I would meet my mentor—someone with the same passion for words as me.

I met Joan for the first time in late October of my sophomore year after school. I had just starting driving and took my time driving from Centerburg to Gambier—the open road still a little unfamiliar to me. She invited me to a seminar that started around four-thirty, so I had time to get something to eat before entering a college class and listening to a woman who would change everything for me.

When I arrived, the seminar was open to the public and there were refreshments in the lobby to bide time while everyone waited for Joan to arrive. I was not sure what she would be talking about or even what she looked like, but I took my seat and waited in the crowd of college students. While waiting, I began to notice the crowd of the room. It seemed that there were only ladies filling the seats talking amongst themselves. Eventually I realized I was the only guy in the room. As nervous tensions started to build at the entire female crowd, the lights dimmed and Joan was introduced to the class and the seminar on woman's rights began.

It was an interesting experience sitting in a room, not knowing a soul, amongst women, as they discussed the woman's liberation movement. No one seemed to much mind a male was among their midst; they probably thought I was the kid of one of the attendees or was told to sit in as a project for another class. I just sat, kept quite and waited for the end—prayed for the end. After about an hour Joan wrapped things up and finished the seminar. As people were filing out, I waited for the crowd to clear a bit and walked up to the podium where she was engaged in a couple of closing conversations before she left.

As I approached she interrupted her conversation, smiled and walked towards me. She stuck out her hand and introduced herself. She had seen me in the crowd as she spoke and figured I was the person she would be mentoring with for next couple of years. She asked for a few moments to say goodbye to the remaining attendees, and then we went back to her office in the Biology building—getting to know each other on the way over.

During this initial meeting we spent most of the time just getting to know one another. She showed me around the labs in which she taught; we talked about her books, and we discussed what it was I was hoping to get out of this experience. After an hour of talking about nothing particular, just feeling each other out, we shook hands and went home for the evening. We had hit it off very well and decided to meet on a regular basis twice a week after school to start digging into the world of authorship and creative writing.

The insights I would gain during those evenings working with Joan would change everything for me. She was exposing me to a world of professional writing that I was not getting in school. I was obtaining a practical education through her, while I received the theoretical education in high school. When she read a short story of mine, she saw the flaws with my work I was not able to see. She told me she had some ideas about what the problems were with my work and I cringed. I had worked so hard to make it as perfect as possible before I gave it to her to read. When she told me it had problems, meaning more than one thing wrong, my heart sank into my stomach. Maybe I was not as good as I thought. Maybe my stories were not as scary as I thought, but I entered her office with my head up and sat across from her waiting to hear all the bad news she had for me.

As she started she told me I had a pretty wild imagination and had the ability to get what was in my head out onto paper in a way by which people could see the images floating through my imagination. With that said, she told me I would have to step out of the box in order to really move the reader, to really scare them. The box? I had no idea what she was talking about, and she knew this by the confused look on my face as I looked at the story I had written lying on her desk. I did not have a clue as to what box my story was in. Hopefully she would be able to get me out of it.

She had also read *A Murder Story* before we met, and she did a comparison between it and the short story I had given her to read. She asked me to make a list of the differences between the two stories. With her help I came up with several differences. The story, the length, the grammar, character development, and so on. When we came to style, she stopped me. *A Murder Story* was written in my early teens and a reader could easily tell the story was written by a young writer, while the short story had a more refined, educated style.

Before the end of the meeting she did not tell me what the box was—this would be something I would learn over several sessions with her. Instead of giving me the answers, she gave me a list of books to read. Together we would read these books, and then discuss them in regards to the various points on the list we had created when we compared my two stories. I would learn what the box was and how to get out of it as we looked at the books we read together.

I left that evening with a list of books to pick up the library, and a mission to figure out what the box was and why my stories were in them. I did not realize as I pursued the mystery of the box, I would learn a life lesson that I would carry with me for the rest of my life. Joan would open a world of possibilities to me through a practical understanding of the world and what the readers sought when they dove into the pages of a good book.

After several more meetings and reading many books, many of them from the past and some from modern writers, I started to see the box around my work. *A Murder Story*, though written by the boy of my past with little understanding in story telling, was a better story then the short story I had given her. It was also better than *Awakening*. I knew it was a more gripping story but was not able to put my finger on why. *Awakening* had a better story line, the characters were more developed, but *A Murder Story* seemed to flow like a poem.

More books were read and analyzed. I was getting closer to seeing the biggest flaw in my new work. Joan helped me along with my discoveries by asking questions. She wanted to know why Shakespeare was so hard to read when compared to Dickens. She asked why Vern was harder to read then King. These were all great writers. They all touched the world in some way, but each was different. Each was from a different era and it was reflected in the way they told the story.

The light finally went on. The difference between the two works I had completed was the way I told the story. *A Murder Story* was written at a time when I did not have a complete understanding of the English language. I wrote the story as if I was telling a group of people around a campfire. It was written truly for my audience. *Awakening* had the barriers of my English class. The stringent rules of correct grammar and form took precedence over the story. I had sterilized the tale of gore I was trying to use to entertain people. It read more like a textbook then a campfire tale. I was so wrapped up in understanding the mechanics of creating the story; I had forced it into a box of rules that did not work when writing for entertainment purposes.

People in general don't speak according to all the rules of proper grammar and do not want to read something where they feel like they need a dictionary to understand its meaning. An audience wants something that flows in the language they speak. Words written on a page used to tell a story should be able to be read out load and have the feel of an everyday conversation.

Joan had shown me I was not lacking in the fundamentals of language, I was over using them. I was trying to be too perfect and the story was suffering from perfection. After I rewrote the short story, keeping in mind the rules of English did not have to always be applied to convey my point, it rivaled *A Murder Story*. Through a series of many essays and short stories, I refined the skill of telling a story using the rules of grammar to support my ideas, not confine them. I went back to telling a story as if people where listing to me as I spoke.

I gained many insights from her during those two years I studied under her, but the most profound was the box. She assured me the creativity was in me to write, and that I had the spirit of a writer, but I had let the story come out they way it was meant to come out. I had to let the paper be my audience and the pen my voice. With this I would be able to convey any story to any reader in a way that would keep the flow of the story moving and bring the reader deep into the frightening world of my mind.

Once the box had been removed, we moved on to deeper elements of a great story, including character development, flow, descriptions, etc. With her I was able to open my mind and creativity to the pen and paper. Many ideas came out and each time they did, they were better than the previous. She was the best thing to happen to me as a writer. Though it would be many years before I would ever see anything of mine printed again, her coaching set the stage for the many novels I have completed and am looking forward to getting them to press for the world to read.

Sometimes a hands on education is the best type in understanding. Some ideas can only be taught in theoretical form in the classroom. It takes real world experience to truly learn those ideas. Working with Joan gave me a real world understanding of the dream I was pursuing. I did not have to throw out the rules and principles I was learning in the classroom, but I did have to put it into perspective when it came to writing the great American novel. With her help I was able to do just that.

30

Theater and Film Passion

Meeting with my mentor on a weekly basis gave me a passion for not only writing but for other avenues within the arts. The Christmas of my sophomore year, I was given a video camera. The camera was another way for me to get the stories floating in my head to the outside world. Pen and paper had been more than adequate, but now I had a visual way to achieve the same goal.

I am not sure why I received the camera that year. Mom had opened herself up to the idea of her son being a horror story teller, but she did not like anything to do with movies. Her hope of seeing me behind a pulpit was still in the back of her mind. Writers could be great preachers, but filmmakers could almost certainly not be a man of God. Those who used the camera's eye were, in her mind, filled with dreams contrary to the principles God had set out for His people. I had asked for a video camera, but did not expect to receive it. To my surprise it was in my stocking hanging over the fireplace Christmas morning.

I now had a toy that would allow me to play out my ideas before a lens to see how they would possibly work on paper. The camera also gave me some great experience in writing dialog that would sound natural to those hearing it spoken. Dialog had been a weak point for me until I had a way of trying it out and listening to it for myself; determining, if what I was trying to say was actually being conveyed in a believable manor.

When I asked why she had given it to me, Mom explained I seemed so happy when I was working with the Mount Vernon Players theater group; she felt it would be another way I would be able to explore the theater bug that had bit me. People had video taped the plays I was in, but for the first time, I would be able to have someone video my own copy of the play. I would be able to see for myself how I was doing.

As I played with the camera to see what I could do, I soon became very proficient at editing multiple takes and making mini movies out of the footage I had shot. It eventually bled over into many school projects and just enhanced my love of film. It fit into the dreams I had to become a writer. I could now film the stories I had written. Film made sense to me and was incorporated into the dreams I had for my life.

The video camera became the third piece to the puzzle of my life and life long goals. I had started to work for the Memorial Theater in Mount Vernon to be closer to and be involved in all the local theater productions. I had also joined the Mount Vernon Players and belonged to a drill team out of Ohio State. I was now developing my skills at writing; I was learning the art of acting and performing, and I was being exposed to a creative medium that would literally allow for anything I could image.

Before receiving the camera, I spent my time at Kenyon with Joan or dong something within the theater group in which I belonged. I had finally found something I was good at and enjoyed doing. While many of my high school friends were playing sports or attending some kind of academic event, I was busy memorizing my lines or spending time on sets getting them ready for the production. I had friends in high school, but the friends I made outside of school were truly my friends. Theater people have their own way of doing things, and they look at life in a very specific way. I fit right in and had many good times and late nights in front of spot lights or at after production parties.

I was exposed to the stage through a class at Centerburg High at the very beginning of my sophomore year. Mrs. Reilly taught theater and debate class that encouraged the development of the performing arts. Through her, the stage soon became a home for me. She would also be the first teacher since my freshman year that would actually see and read my own work. In her English class during my junior year, I had decided to stop copying for others and started submitting my own work. I had not written anything for school for two years, but she encouraged originality no matter what the content.

Through one of the productions at Centerburg High, I was introduced to a group of people who worked for the Memorial Theater on a regular basis. By meeting them, I met a way to get involved in theater outside the rules and restrictions of a public school system. It was not long before I was offered a job after school to help out around the theater as a stage and technical hand. This now became a place of exploration and introduced me to many people with the same aspirations and dreams.

While working at the theater, I met people from all over the country. I was exposed to other acting and dance groups, and it was not long before I became a member of a drill team/production group out of Columbus. They were located on the Ohio State campus and had access to all kinds of materials to enhance our productions. They also had access to the assistance of the Ohio State theatrical staff that knew all the tricks of trade and were more than willing to share their ideas and talents with the group.

Over a three year period, I would spend my evenings with my mentor, at the Memorial Theater, in Columbus with my drill team, or learning as much as I could about the performing arts through the professionals at Ohio State. I built an entire life for myself outside of high school. The people I had grown up with were becoming less and less a part of my life. I was building something outside the walls of Centerburg High and was having a great time doing it. I had begun to touch the world and was looking forward to the day when I would be out and able to explore everything I could imagine without the hindrance of high school.

By the time I made into my junior year, I had become completely immersed in my writing, learning to use my video camera, and enjoying my nights filled with dance performances and stage productions. Other student's had sports or the band and choir or some other school activity; I had the arts. Though Mom and Dad never came to any of the productions I was involved in, Mom gave me the freedom to seek out the dreams of my teens. She had become immersed in church. I was there every Sunday and she was happy with that. As long as I was in the pew during service, she felt she still had a chance to get me behind the pulpit.

In my family, each had something to keep them occupied and out of the others way. David was spending time with his friends, I was out working on a stage, and Mom had her church groups. We all had our own outlets tailored to each of us, keeping us out of each other's way while maintaining a balance at home that kept many of the problems of a growing household out at the curb.

31

MTV High

When my junior year was coming to an end, I had to make a choice about what I wanted out of school. Centerburg was not giving me the flexibility I needed to continue pursuing the things I found most important in life. Centerburg was simply too small to accommodate the needs I had for a school and after school activities. I needed to go someplace that would allow me to take the next step after maxing out the resources offered at Centerburg.

At first, I looked to go towards Columbus for my studies. The high schools there were accustomed to dealing with students who had special interests, but none of them fit into my schedule. They were all too far from Kenyon College and the Memorial Theater where I worked. They were closer to the activities I had in Columbus, but it would mean I would have to give up some of the obligations I had right after school. I simply did not have the time to drive from Columbus back into Mount Vernon. I would be too far away.

Mom had some concerns about me leaving the school I had grown up in when I was so close to graduation, but when she looked at what I was doing after school and my reasons for leaving, she finally came aboard, but she would make the final decision as to where I would go.

Mom had noticed friends from Centerburg never came by the house for visits. They were always people from Kenyon or the theater groups I was involved with. She knew the girls I dated where from different schools. For my junior prom I went to Fredericktown's instead of Centerburg's. High school had simply become a place where I went to get through school. I had a few friends while I was there, but my real friends were from other places. So leaving Centerburg was nothing more then transferring where I took my classes during the day. I wasn't leaving my friends or a place where I had great involvement. I was simply moving to another school to further myself. The rest of my life would remain unchanged. I would still have the same friends and be going to same places in the evenings.

In May of my junior year, I decided to transfer to Mount Vernon High for my senior year. I am not even sure why I did not just decide to go there in the beginning when I started looking. I had been there several times doing things with their theater group and knew a lot of people in attendance. I had also spent many evenings there with others who were involved in the mentoring program. The school board tried to get us together at least a couple of times a month so we could discuss how things were going and so forth. So MTV High was not something new to me. They also offered everything I wanted and was close enough to Kenyon and my work to allow me to keep my schedule after school.

For Mom, Mount Vernon kept me close to home instead of driving thirty miles one way for high school. I did not have to do much convincing; before I even finished my junior year at Centerburg, I was already enrolled at Mount Vernon for the next year. This would be the school where I would graduate and call my high school home. I left Centerburg and everything I knew with less than ten minutes worth of paperwork and a handshake with my new counselor. It was not a hard decision for me. I was simply replacing one set of rules and classes, for another that more suited what I needed.

On the last day of school during my junior year, I said goodbye to the old brick building I had called home during the day and reached for something new with new people. During the summer I went through a small orientation and scheduled my classes. While in orientation I was asked if I wanted to help out in the athletic department. They needed a sports medic to do some of the more basic activities while the certified medics focused their attention to more pressing issues with the athletes. I took the opportunity as a way to meet more people in my new school. I only knew a few of the other students and this would allow me to meet others before school started. I would be able to work with the soccer teams, volleyball team, and football team during the day.

Until this summer, I knew very little about sports. I had always been attracted to the arts. I had never been to a football game or basketball game while I attended Centerburg, but that was all about to change. I would learn the rules of every sport Mount Vernon offered and became an instant sports fan, something I thought would never happen. I guess it just took the right exposure to get me involved in something that had never interested me in the past.

As time went by, I became very proficient at taping ankles, bandaging cuts, and reducing swelling. I also began to have an understanding of the sports world I had never had before. I used to change the channel when football or basketball was on, but I now found myself watching and understanding, even enjoying myself. I can honestly say Mount Vernon and the friends I made there made me a fan of the Steelers and Buccaneers, the Pistons and the Magic, and the Red Wings and Penguins. They opened a world to me that had once been a mystery. This brought me into a world I was always looking in on but never able to be a part of. Now I had my teams. I had someone to root for during play offs, even though my choice in teams was not always the best. I will always be a fan, and have grown greatly simply by being one.

My senior year spent at Mount Vernon High School turned out to be the best year of my high school life. Like moving to a new town or starting a new job, I was able to redefine myself. The other students of Mount Vernon did not know who I was, giving me the opportunity to impress upon them the image I wanted instead of what was given to me during the many years at Centerburg. I could be whoever I wanted to be.

It took a while, but eventually I blended into the senior class without notice. I was a senior at Mount Vernon High, and no one could tell I had only been there for a year. I was just like everyone else who had started from Kindergarten. This would be my last year spent in high school, and I am proud to say I spent it at MTV high. It provided for me everything I needed and expected and has become a cherished memory of the past.

32

The Average American Family

As I started my senior year of high school, life was good for my family. My mother, through hard work and sacrifice, had done what most can only dream of doing. She had left her family and her childhood life behind, and started fresh, with the only option that of success. Failure was something that was not possible. Failure to her meant falling short as a woman and as a mother to her two children, and that would not happen. She had done whatever it took, and then some, to ensure she succeeded.

With only a high school education, she worked herself through the ranks of Nationwide, creating for herself a foundation of security build on the years of tireless work and effort. She had done what many had thought impossible and many had even hoped to see her fail.

I had started to venture out into the world to see what was out there, and I found there was so much more than the little town we lived in. I dreamed of becoming a great horror writer and film director. Everything was going well in my life. When I look back I see this time as a period in my life when absolutely anything was possible. I just had to reach out and take it. I dreamed of film school after high school and wrote constantly in the hopes of creating the next Freddy Kruger, Jason Voorhees, or Michael Myers. I wanted to sit behind the camera and capture the horrors of my imagination in hopes of keeping little children up at night after sneaking out to watch one of my movies.

All of this was possible then. I could have anything I wanted. Mount Vernon High School would be the first step I would take into the depths of change the world required in order to follow the dreams of the heart. I was starting my journey to a future I longed to become the present. I could hardly wait for what was lying ahead of me.

Even David was becoming his own man in the adult world. He was building a life with his friends and starting to look beyond the horizon at what might be possible. Life was no longer the play ground of the past, but an infinite amount of possibilities that he was just starting to realize. As he watched my first steps forward, he began to long for the time when he would be able step out and explore the world.

The three of us lived in Centerburg, Ohio, and considered this small town in the middle of the state home. Lynchburg was nothing to David and I, and we considered ourselves Yankees just like our friends. Even Mom had lost her touch with her past life. She remained in contact with those from her other life, but they were merely reflections of those she once thought of as family. Her sisters and aunts and uncles, where now living in Ohio. They may not have been blood relatives, but they became her family and the family of her two children.

It could be easily said, we were the average American family. We lived in small town America in a ranch house on a couple of acres of land among the corn and soy fields. There was always a family dog roaming the yard and past times were filled with dirt bike riding and hanging out with friends. David and I went to school where we knew everyone and everyone knew us. Driving through town required nods and waves to the people passing by or those whom you saw out in their yards or at the gas station. We waved to our friends, and they were everywhere throughout the small town.

Our Sundays were filled with church, and our weeks were spent at school. Life had become a routine that many can only dream of having. Who really does not want to live someplace where everyone knows your name and has a hand of support reached out when you need it? I have not met anyone who when asked, and really thinks about the question, does not desire to belong to a community. Everyone wants this, and I had it. I belonged to Centerburg as much as the mayor, the local real estate agent, or any of my friends. This was home.

Pure happiness and joy only lasts moments in our lives. These moments are the very driving force of life. Everything we do in life is to recapture the feeling of waking up Christmas morning at age four and seeing Santa had visited, of receiving our first kiss, falling in love for the first time. These moments are what make the obstacles worth over coming. Years of pain are worth just a moment of pure joy. Our ambitions in life are to get just a taste of this feeling.

Just like everyone else in life, my few moments of indescribable, pure happiness where about to come to an end, only to be followed by years of failure after failure and heartaches so deep they threatened to destroy the person I had once been. I was looking to the future and seeing film school, published novels, but what awaited was a black cloud that would last for years.

My family had greatness in the love we had for one another, the drive each of us had to succeed, and the bright futures all of us hoped would pan out, but just like any other family a cloud was starting to form and the bubble of happiness would soon be popped, exposing us all to the darker side of the world around us.

PART III
Closure to the Past

33

August 1994

At the beginning of August, 1994, I was readying myself for my senior year at Mount Vernon High School. I had spent most of the summer working with the football team during the day and working for the theater in the evenings. A trip to the beach and a trip to Cedar Point broke the summer monotony, but it was mostly spent working.

One afternoon after coming home for bandaging cuts and wrapping ankles for the team, I received a call from Mom to hang out for a while. She needed to talk with David and I. I argued that I had to get to the theater as soon as possible; opening night was just a few days away and there was still a lot of work to be done. After a few moments of protest, I told her I would be home, and David would be with me waiting for her to get there.

I took my shower; got everything I needed for work ready and waited for Mom to come home. It was around noon when she called which meant she was leaving work early. The last time she had left early from work and asked for me to be home when she got there was when her dad had died. She had left work early and told David and I our grandfather had died and that we would be going to Lynchburg for the funeral services. I can remember seeing her come home with her best friend Mary and sitting David and I down in the kitchen to tell us the news. She needed Mary more so for herself than she did for David and I.

It was not long before Mom's car pulled into the driveway, Mary in the passenger seat. As they got out and walked up sidewalk, seeing the two of them together coming here to talk to David and I filled me with a sense of dread. I was trying to figure out who had died, but I could not think of anyone close who was sick. The only person I could think of who may have died was Ida, a close friend of the family from the church. She had been fighting cancer for some time, but it was looking like the treatments were working. Ida was up and around and looked as if her battle with cancer was over. Whatever the news, it was bad by the expressions on their faces, and the very fact Mary was needed to support Mom while she told us whatever news they had.

When they came in, I was told to get David and sit in the living room. Mary made small talk, asking how things were going while Mom went to the bathroom. I had long forgotten about the obligations I had to the theater production; I just wanted to know who had died. Who was I going to being visiting at a funeral home and mourning their loss. Not knowing was worse then actually finding out. The sooner I knew, the sooner I could deal with the dreaded news. Thinking about the possibilities was creating an internal hysteria that could only be eased by whatever the two of them where going to tell my brother and I.

A few moments went by while we waited for Mom to finish her business in the bathroom and join us in the living room, waiting to hear whatever it was she had to say. She sat in the chair across from David and I on the sofa. Before she could speak, her words were cut off by the tears she had been holding back since she walked through the front door. Whatever the news was, when she looked at the two of us, it became unbearable to her.

Mary put her arm around her for comfort as David and I waited in horror. Watching her breakdown was worse than the wait for the news. She was always so strong, but she was not able to deal with news she had to give us. Before I had received the phone call from her that day, everything was going very well, but she now held something that would change everything in my life and in my brother's life. This news would not be about the passing of a loved one, it was going to be something worse; something that would have an affect on my entire family.

I had been told, and had even started to experience, that life did not always work out the way it was planned, but never had I been exposed to the really harsh realities of life until this moment. I had read many books about people making one mistake or having an accident and how those very quick events in their lives changed everything for the individual, sometimes for the best but often for the worse.

Life became very real to me as Mom dried her eyes and told David and I she had breast cancer. Not only did she have cancer, but she had one of the most aggressive and damaging forms known. Through teary eyes she explained her chances of recovering were not very good and that the doctors had given her a half year to a full year to live, even with rigorous treatment.

For once I had nothing to say. She asked if either of us had any questions, but neither David nor I asked. We did not even know what we should be asking. We had just been told our mother was going to die. This was a third of our family; she was the point on the pyramid of our lives. What could we ask? I have cancer and have at most a year to live, summed up everything for the two of us. We already knew she had looked into all of her options. Mom knew what she was facing and gave us the news after exhausting hope to make it through.

Seeing our blank looks and gaining control of herself, she told us what her plan would be for the next year. She briefly told us about the mastectomy she would be having and then subsequent chemotherapy and radiation treatments. She promised us she would fight. She looked at my brother and I and told us everything would be alright. God would take care of us. He would make sure things worked out for the best. God was where she put her hopes in beating the disease, but as I looked at her and thought about what lay ahead, I did not see God.

I was not entirely sure what lay ahead as my family moved through the months fighting cancer, but I could not see God anywhere in the future. I was starting to see death and failure, not peace and happiness. Mortality started to become a realization of life, and the security I had once felt in my home was beginning to crumble. This afternoon would be the beginning of a long road, filled with tremendous failure, unbearable loss, and years of struggle.

When it was over, Mom looked at her two sons and knew we had heard her words but did not understand the implications of what was going to happen. In less than fifteen minutes our lives had changed forever. It would take months for the information to sink in and an understandability to develop between my brother and I.

When she was done, she told me to get off to work before I was too late to help out, and told David he could go out with his friends for the evening. Mary and her retired to the kitchen to have coffee.

David left to be with his friends, and I went to the theater to get some work done before the show in a few days. I did not work very long; I cut out early to have dinner with Samantha. It was probably better that I left early. I was not being much help, and it was good to spend some time with Sam. She and I had started to date a few weeks before and being with her took my mind off the bombshell from earlier in the evening.

I did not get home until late that night, sometime around midnight, but Mom was still up. I was fairly certain she would still be up when I got home. Usually she would have been in bed before ten so she could get up early the next morning for work, but tonight, I knew she wanted to talk with me. I had stayed out later than usual that night hoping she would have given up and gone to bed for the night. I was not ready for the conversation we would be having. I knew I would eventually have to talk with her about the future of the family, but I was not ready that night.

When I pulled into the drive, I saw the living room light still on and almost backed back out and went to a friend's house for the night, but I could not help thinking about her sitting in her chair waiting for her oldest son to come home. She wanted to talk to her son, and I did not want to disappoint her. The news was hard to deal with, but I could not imagine what it was like for her. She had been told she would die. She had been told, everything she had worked so hard for, had left behind, had been for nothing. She would never be able to enjoy the fruits of the years of hard work.

I went in, and she had cake waiting in the kitchen. She never could cook so the cake was store bought, but it was the best cake I had ever had. We stayed up late into the night talking about everything in our lives; nothing was off the table in the discussion.

I knew my mother well enough to know she had known about the tumors for some time. I could tell by the way she had broken down when she told David and I. That would not have happened if there was hope of recovery, which meant she had known and had looked into treatment options way before my brother and I even knew there was a problem.

Roughly six months prior she had felt a lump on her breast while getting ready for work and went to the doctor to have it looked at. It was found that original lump was a cyst caused by to much caffeine. Mom was working a full time load at work and was going to school full time in the evening. Coffee and its caffeine had become a great friend of hers.

The news was very comforting to her and the cyst did go down after she had reduced her coffee intake. It was also a wake up call to her. She was pushing herself too hard. Working and going to school full time was just too much. She was not in her early twenties anymore. Her body could not cope with the added stress over long periods of time like it once could.

Everything seemed to be going well. The original lump had all but gone away, and she had more energy after cutting back on her school load. Instead of going full time, she went to school on the weekends part-time. Just like before, she was getting ready for work when she felt another lump. This time the lump did not turn out to be a benign cyst, but a tumor intent on spreading. In a six month period, she had gone from being healthy to dying. There were no other warnings, just the lump felt after it was too late.

Mom tried to explain to me what was going to happen next as far as treatment and surgery went, but she was just as unsure as I was. Neither of us had gone through anything like this before. We both knew a couple of people from church and our former neighbor who had cancer, but neither of us had actually been through the really gritty parts of the ordeal. These were roads we had heard about but had never traveled.

That morning I had awoken to a world where anything was possible, but I went to bed that night with the noose of life around my neck. From this day forward, I would awaken to a world with it around my neck and feel it steadily get tighter.

I am not sure when she told her family back in Lynchburg, but I know Dad knew roughly the same time David and I were told. He came up that weekend to get the details and to face the reality of losing the woman he had loved but never could live with. I did not see the relationship they had until that weekend. I did not understand why neither of them ever remarried, but I saw it as I watched them sitting around the kitchen table. They were divorced but still husband and wife in their minds. They did not live together, but still loved one another as if they were still on their honeymoon. Together, they were a paradox I was just beginning to understand.

34

Senior Year Begins

My senior year started with some very rough bumps, but I was looking forward to the first day of school. During the summer I had put in a lot of the time with the Mount Vernon High soccer team, football team, and volleyball team. During my work as an assistant sports medic, I made several new friends and knew many of the people I would be going to school with.

Meeting people and having friends was something I thought would have been an issue after leaving Centerburg High. I had not grown up with this senior class, but when the first period bell rang, I was sitting in my Physics class with several friends. It took less than one day for me to feel as if I had grown up with this group, Centerburg High now something foreign to me.

Just before that first day of my last year of high school, Mom's sister Wanda came to visit. She had come not only for a visit but for my mother's first surgery. The shock of the news of the cancer had worn off, but the apprehension and fear was still evident in everyone involved. The mastectomy was the first step in a long process Mom would have to endure before her ordeal would be over. Having Wanda by her side gave Mom a comforting face to look upon and a sister's ear to listen to her.

The mastectomy did not take long. The cancer was only in one breast. The real fear was not the cancer in the breast but how much, if any, had spread to her interior chest lining. No one would be able to tell any of us how much the cancer had spread until the surgery was over. When the doctors came in to check on her recovery progress, my brother and I, her sister, our dad, everyone involved, waited to hear if the cancer was spreading.

The oncologist said the surgery went very well, most of the tumors had been removed. The remaining parts of the cancer were in the chest lining, but treatments had a good chance of preventing further spreading and possibly pushing the cancer into remission. Mom's doctors had given all of us a little hope. The possibility of chemotherapy and radiation working was something for all of us to hold on to. Instead of the looming fear of death in a year, hope of many years of life now started to fill our souls.

I had thought I would start my first day of school knowing that this would be the last year I would have with my mother, but instead I started with the expectation she would be around to see me graduate from college. I knew she had cancer and the year ahead of me would be tough, but at least there was some light at the end of the tunnel.

The first few weeks of my senior year at my new school went far better than I could have anticipated. I was doing well academically, and my evenings were filled with working with the soccer and football teams and the theater. Mom spent the time recovering from her surgery and gearing herself up for the chemotherapy that would soon start.

For the first time since we had moved to Ohio, Mom was spending most of her time at home. She had taken medical leave from work while she had her breast removed and the ports for the treatments placed into her chest. She used the time between her surgeries and the start of her chemo to get herself ready for the impending hair loss and the lack of one breast. She purchased a wig that matched her natural hair and hair style and bought a silicon replacement to fill the empty space on her chest.

She had no intention of staying away from work any longer than she absolutely had to—there was simply too much to be done. Once her treatments started, she expected to work in between them, taking off just enough time to recover from the massive dose of chemicals in her system.

When it was time for Mom's first treatment, Wanda was still around to help out with her care after treatment. David and I kept ourselves busy at school, while Mom recuperated at home. None of us knew what the treatments were going to do to my mother. We just knew that chemo tended to make the patient sick, lose their hair, and made them very weak for a couple of days after. Wanda stayed to see how things were going to go and David and I made sure the house stayed in order.

The chemotherapy made Mom sick for just a few days after her first treatment. Mainly nauseous, she got up every morning, got dressed, and made an effort to have a routine day. It did not take long until she was ready to go back to work. Just days after being pumped full of chemicals, she went back to work like everything was going as it always had.

With her doing so well, Wanda went back home. She could not stay in Ohio indefinitely; she had a family back in Lynchburg to care for. With Mom handling the treatments so well, there was no need for her to hang around. Before leaving, she told David and I she was just a phone call away and not to ever hesitate to call.

Just at the start of October, our home started to get back to normal. People were not roaming in and out as much to see how Mom was doing. Mom had gone back to work until her next treatment at the end of the month, and David and I were completely involved in our own activities. Dad had gone back to Virginia soon after the mastectomy, but would be returning for my birthday on the eleventh of October. Before he returned, Mom took me out to dinner to have a talk with me. This would be the first of many talks we would have about what lay ahead and what needed to be done in order to keep our lives together. These talks were nothing like the sex and drugs talks; they went far deeper and had a far more reaching impact on my perception of my life.

Over a steak diner, she told me I had to make an effort to make it right between Dad and I. The problems we were having could no longer continue. There simply was not enough time for them to work themselves out with Mom as the mediator. She told me there was a good possibility she would not be around much longer and that the rifts between Dad and I needed to be closed. While she was talking, I heard for the first time, from her mouth, in her own words, she would not live forever. Everyone knows their parents are not going to be their forever, but this was the first time I truly realized she was going to be gone soon.

She continued to talk, but all I could think of was her eventual death. The problems between Dad and I were no longer important—just her admission of looming death. Before this dinner between mother and son, God was always the one in control, and Mom had faith in God to make her well. She never lost that faith, but she faced reality and was preparing for the worse.

Mom must have noticed I was still hung up on her death and not paying attention to the issue with Dad. She stopped herself and explained to me there were things she needed to tell me before it was too late. Most parents have the opportunity of time in order to tell their children about family secrets, explain the realities of life, and help their children through their learning period into adulthood. She was not sure how much time she had and wanted to do what she could to help when she was gone.

After getting my attention, I agreed to make a conscious effort to make things right between Dad and I. I would not go out of my way to avoid him, but instead, try to make him a part of my life. With that agreement, the rest of the dinner was filled with more pleasant conversations about the girl I was dating, how school was going, and what I was up to in the theater and at dance class. She talked about work and church, and both of us were able to laugh a bit. Our differences of the past were not brought up. They seemed to be so distant and no where near as important as they had once seemed.

It was a perfect dinner—one I will never forget. It would be the last time she would look like the mother of my youth. She still had her hair and was still very healthy looking, but the next time we met to have a dinner between just the two of us, the ravages of cancer would start to be evident.

35

God, A Hopeless Hope

From the very moment I was told Mom had cancer, I was told God would see everything through. God would bless the family according to His will. Along with the potential for the treatments to send the cancer into remission, there was also the power of God. I was told, through Him anything could be accomplished or overcome, but soon found faith in God was no more effective then a child's faith in Santa to make Christmas the best holiday of the year.

The cancer just strengthened Mom's faith, but it began to expose the realities of God and His erratic ways of running the world and helping those who sought Him for help and guidance. Mom was confident her savior Jesus was beside her the entire time she was sick, but I was the one lifting her head from her pillow so she could vomit into the trash can. I was left to deal with what He had done.

The first couple of treatment with Mom had went pretty well. The recovery time between treatments was relatively short, but it soon lengthened to a point where Mom could hardly take care of herself. As she praised the ways of her Lord, I watcher her wither into nothing. Once a strong woman, she was now reduced to hardly being able to go to the bathroom.

My nights were now filled with the stark sounds of gagging as Mom dry heaved, coughed, and moaned from the aches in her joints from the effects of chemotherapy. She would lay in her bed for days before having the strength to get up and sit in the living room in her Lay-Z-Boy. The woman who I called Mom, remembering her having a head full of hair and being pleasantly plump, was now completely bald, thinning tremendously, and sluggish with pain. Her God had failed her.

God allowed those who did wicked things to get shot, or have a heart attack, or killed in a car accident. He gave them a quick death, something that truly is a blessing. No one wants to linger in agony. Everyone wants to go quickly, but with God, only the damned were blessed with the mercy of dying instantly. For His followers, He had a sadistic way of lengthening the pain of passing on.

I was told by the pastor of our church, God did this to test the faith of His people, that everything was a part of His divine plan, and faith would see us all through. This made no sense to me. People are always the most faithful when the going gets tough. Faith during a time of crisis was simply something done out of desperation. Faith during the good times is a much better test of devotion.

Seeing God was nothing more then a distant entity, if He even existed, was enough for me to push Him to the side and put my hopes and dreams on the shoulders of humanity. God was not a player in my life, and I was not going to waste anymore of my time on Him. I stopped going to church, and stopped supporting the ways of God. His ways had brought my family and I nothing but suffering, and the worst was yet to come. God was punishing my mother for serving Him. She did not smoke, drink, keep late nights, or any other habit of a wild life. She had sought His guidance and was lead to her death.

Mom was guilty of working hard, raising her children to the best of her ability, and serving her God in every conceivable way she could. For this, a plague was placed in my house hold. The people of the faith told me it was all in God's plan and that it was happening for the betterment of everyone involved. God was doing this to help invigorate my family to a greater faith in His holy promise.

While they spoke, giving ambiguous explanations, I was learning touching God and anything to do with Him was like touching a hot stove. After laying a bare hand on the glowing burner, one learned quickly not to touch it again. God was my searing burner, and I quickly learned it was dangerous to get to close.

Just looking at my mother's life, I could see hard work and determination made a person's life, determined how well they did in life. She had overcome insurmountable obstacles to provide great things to David and I, and she had done it without God. She only turned to Him when the task was done, the achievements achieved. She seemed to have already learned, you get burned if you put your faith in God.

An hour on ones knees praying was wasted time. That hour could be used for far more constructive activities, such as cleaning the house, putting in overtime at work, spending time with loved ones, or helping someone else overcome the obstacles in their lives.

Mom watched as I wondered from the faith she so desperately tried to instill in my brother and I. She now took it onto herself to push God at me and do everything she could to guild me in a direction she and God had planned out for my life. With this new push, the fights of my early teens again came back into play in our lives.

The arguments over writing horror, dance class, and theater had never really been resolved. We had just worked out a way to keep it away from each other. Mom did not go to any of the plays or dance performances and certainly did not read anything I wrote, and I went to church every Sunday. Each of us did what we wanted and life seemed to move on without incident. But with me not going to church and not seeking the healing power of the Lord, the balance had been tipped, and she was going to do everything to make it balanced again, if not tipped in God's favor.

The steadiness and understanding we had between the two of us quickly dissolved. Years earlier I had been convinced God was real and active in our lives, but I could see through her own actions and the statements and remarks of the members of our church, that God was nothing more then a hope created in a time before humanity was able to provide for itself. Man looked to the supernatural for guidance instead of what they saw before them.

God was created in order to understand the world when human knowledge fell short. As knowledge increased, the Godly mysteries were understandable and a piece of God was no more. Today people still turn to God when understanding is in short supply instead of looking for the true answers to the questions and problems of their lives.

I did not have a problem with Mom believing in these frivolous dreams, but I was not going to fall into the trap of holding on to an impossible hope. I put my faith in the accomplishments of hard work and dedication. There seemed to be a far greater chance of success than praying to an empty God.

From here on I was determined not to be trapped into the illusions of faith. My life would be determined by the work I put into it. No longer would I see my mistakes as the will of God, but my own short comings, learn from them and move on. I will make, and have made, many bad decisions in my life, but they were my choices.

If God was unwilling to help my mother after following His lead, then I would not have anything to do with Him anymore. Following a leader who led His people off a bridge was not something I would do with my life. Even if I failed at the many challenges ahead of me, at least I would not suffer the heart break of being abandoned by the very God I once held in such regard.

At the age of eighteen, I left God to the memories of my childhood and looked forward to a life undetermined by a malevolent deity.

36

Dad

After being convinced by Mom that the relationship between Dad and I needed to be amended, I began spending time with the man in hopes of finding a common ground. For the last several years, we had spent most of our time avoiding each other, but now we were being thrust into a relationship whether we liked it or not. I stopped being so critical, and he stopped being so demanding on my time. This tenuous blend of him letting go a little and of me not being so harsh on his appearance and mannerisms left just enough room for the two of us to being talking and really begin to get to know one another.

Even if Mom had not insisted we mend the gaps between us, they would have closed on their own as her treatments progressed and her time in the hospital began to lengthen. Though there were people around while Mom fought her cancer, Dad was the only one who would be around after the inevitable. He had been around my entire life for weekends, vacations, and holidays. He would become the constant that would not change for a long time, something I needed in order to look ahead. At least I knew he would be there.

Instead of visiting Mom in the hospital alone, he was always there right beside me in everything that was happening in our family. His presence was enough. Just having him there was a comfort that allowed me to overlook many of the faults that so irked me in the past.

Before now, I really did not know who my Dad was and where he came from. As a boy he had been the one who shared the Star Wars passion with me. He was the one who had supported me while Mom did everything she could to keep me from writing. He was the one who had taken me to the movies, bought me books, and let me stay up late to watch Elvira as she hosted late night horror marathons, but I did not really know him as a person.

By the time I was old enough for him to let down his parental guard, we had parted ways. All we had were the occasional birthday or holiday during my teen years—not enough time for our different personalities to build the bridges of communication. This time in the hospital, or taking care of the house while Mom was undergoing treatment, made up for much of the lost time.

His time serving our country in Vietnam became the conduit that would start to mend the gaps of the past. With Desert Storm and learning about the World Wars and the Korean and Vietnam wars in school, I was interested in what he could tell me about his time spent out in the jungle. When I was in the eighth grade he had pushed hard to ensure I always supported the American troops and showed total respect for the uniforms they wore. Until sitting in the waiting rooms with him waiting for Mom to finish with the doctors, I had not thought about why he had been so adamant about his views. I was finally capable of somewhat understanding what it meant to be a soldier, and he took the opportunity to tell me about his time spent in the Army.

As he talked, I could see how the few years he had spent overseas fighting; returning to a country who hated him for his service, had messed with his mind. He watched as the troops returned from Iraq greeted with open arms—had worked to ensure they returned to a country grateful for their hard work, but was still looking for his thank you. Ever since returning from Vietnam, he was searching for the parade and the attention him and his fellow soldiers deserved.

This longing for attention had been the wedging divide between Mom, myself, and every other person Dad came in contact with in a personal way. Not getting the respect and admiration he deserved for his service, he made up other ways to gain the attention he longed for more than anything in life. If he could not be honored; he would attempt to be pitied by those around him.

These attempts at creating pity would become a sport of sorts with David and I. We found that no matter how bad someone had it in life, Dad had it worse. If Mom had high blood pressure, Dad had several mild heart attacks to top her. If David had muscle cramps from football practice, Dad had muscle cramps from some disease from the jungles. If someone was taking medication, he was taking more. At times, we would just make up stuff to see what he would come up with.

It was a constant battle that he felt he could not loose. He always seemed to feel he had to have a problem in order to have people like him. He never seemed to realize, his fantastic problems were the very reason why people were pushed away. No one wants to be around someone who is always complaining just to get a few minutes consideration.

Eventually, I tired of listening to him ramble on about how bad his health was in comparison to Mom's. I asked him just to let me know if something serious was wrong so that I could get him to the hospital. I did not have to hear about every little problem he was having. I had enough to deal with regarding Mom's condition.

At first he seemed to be hurt that I did not want to know about the numerous fabricated medical conditions he was enduring, but as time passed he realized nothing had changed between the two of us. We still went out to the movies and fishing. He did not need my sympathy to get attention from me; he just had to be there. He just needed to be Dad, nothing else was needed.

It took several months, but the two of us were back on speaking terms with one another, and we started to build new bonds formed by the experiences of the present instead of those of the past. No longer were we looking to the years of my youth to find common ground; we were stepping out onto new ground.

37

Looking For a College

Like every senior in high school, I had the dream of going to college. I could not wait to get out on my own and start exploring the things in which I was truly interested. College was a doorway into another world, something completely different from the institutional environment created by teachers and parents to coddle their children into adulthood.

As the guidance counselors passed out information about college, I already had my mind made up. I was going to film school. It was a dream of mine for as long as I could remember to be a director—to even write the screenplays for the movies I would direct. Finally, I would be able to really explore film. Instead of playing with video cameras after school hours, I would be able to take classes that would teach me the trade and polish my skills while making my dreams come true.

When I brought the applications home to Mom to go over, I hit a brick wall. She would have nothing to do with me going to a film school. She had humored me enough with my dreams of being a writer or directing films. In her mind, it was time for me to get back to reality—to pick a field of study she could be proud to talk about with her church friends. Film was everything she was against, and she would have no part in sending her son to a school that encouraged the movies of our day.

Debating with her did not do much good, and I just dropped the subject with her. I filled the applications out on my own and guessed on the financial aid questions. It was around Christmas when UCLA, Full Sail Film Academy, and New York Film Institute replied to my application. I managed to get into them all. The top three film schools in the world had accepted me into their programs, but the celebration was short.

I was not the one who checked the mail each day. Mom was home and checked the mail each day. When I got home from school, I had to open my letters in front of her, just to have her through them away without any regard to what I wanted when high school was over. I tried to explain to her that Full Sail was considered the Harvard of film schools. It was an honor to be asked to attend—so very few were accepted each year.

The Christmas holiday was filled with my disappointment and her determination to decide the fate of her child. Even with her being so ill, I could hardly stand being in the house with her. I knew that this Christmas could be the last she had with us, but I did whatever I could not to go home. I was afraid I would say something I would not be able to take back or something that would just solidify her determination. Time would be the only thing I could use to convince her to let me go. If a fight broke out over the holiday, it would just ruin the jolly festivities and end all hopes I had of going to film school.

Even though Mom was not on board with my plans for my life, I still pressed forward. The only real obstacle preventing me from going to the school of my choice was money. Financing was the only card Mom had to play when it came to where I went to school. She made to much money for me to receive enough financial aid to pay for school with out her support.

Since federal loans and grants were out of the question, the only avenues left for me were scholarships. I already received an academic scholarship, but I was still several thousand dollars short. It was far more then I would be able to make working while in school. I had to find another way to pay my way.

With the help of the counselors at Mount Vernon High School and the direction of my mentor at Kenyon College, I did find a way. I would be able to work for a film company while in school if I contracted my services to them for a minimum of five years after I graduated. If I did this, they would pay for the remaining tuition and provide a job during my time in school, and of course, I would have a job when I finished.

While I was working so diligently to find a way to pay for school, Mom had taken it upon herself to apply for schools she felt were more suitable to her son's needs. Kenyon College was at the top of her list. She figured I had been going there throughout my high school years so it would be something that was familiar to me and close to home. The others were Otterbein College, Ohio State University, and Liberty University.

She asked me to write the essay each school had requested—she did not really ask, she made me write them, but I made sure they would not accept me. I did not want to go to those schools, and figured if they did not accept me, then she would have to let me go to one of the film schools.

I tried to get denied by all four but two still accepted the essay I wrote. Liberty University and Ohio State both seemed to think the dribble I had sent them was enough. In March I received letters from both schools congratulating me on my acceptance. She knew I tried to blow the application process. When the denial came back from Kenyon College, she called my mentor to see what had happened. Mom was informed the essay submitted was horrendous, well below my abilities. They felt that if I could not take the essay on the application serious then I was not serious about attending. She let me know, even though I had tried, I was still accepted into two schools she would gladly support me in if I attended.

I did not tell her I had found a way to go to film school without her help. I still had a few things to finalize. Mainly, I had to go to the studio for an interview before I could get final approval. Trying to figure out how to get to Orlando without her knowing why I was going would be difficult, but I did not see a reason to get into it with her before I had figured out how to get to that interview.

Dad was the one who stepped up when I needed help. I needed to go to Florida over Spring Break, and he wanted to go. It was my senior year, and the trip to Orlando seemed within reason. Mom packed my bags and we left. While there, I did the interview and was accepted into the work study program. Dad was glad to see I would be able to follow the dream he had supported for the last five years. He had been the one to provide me with books. He bought me my first typewriter, and now his efforts were being realized in my ability.

That trip was the finest time I had with my dad. Everything was perfect as we started back home. I had the financing I needed to go to school, a job guarantee after school, and the opportunity to work in the literary and film industries. My life had been turned inside out with Mom getting cancer, but it now seemed everything would work out. I still had something to strive for and look forward to, but that too would be taken away when we rolled back into Centerburg.

Getting back late after a day of driving, I went right to bed when I got home. I did not unpack the car; I just crawled into bed and went right out. Dad had the pleasure of sleeping for the second part of the drive and was wide awake when we got home. Mom had slept most of the day due the chemo and was up when we got home and offered to make me something to eat. I told her no thank you and went to my room, but Dad sat in the kitchen and talked with Mom for most of the night.

I thought I had everything planned out, but I forgot to tell Dad I had not told Mom about the interview. That night they talked about me going to film school and the entire plan was laid out before Mom. I did not have a chance to grease the wheels; Dad had given it all up before I was ready. My college decision was going to be made sooner than I was expecting.

Dad and I had retuned home late Saturday night. Sunday morning Mom went to church and hurried right home to have a talk with her oldest son. The decision on school would be determined that afternoon, and it would be something that she wanted. She was the parent; I was the child. Her plans for my life were based on life's experiences. Mine were on the whims of hopeful dreams—dreams she felt were inappropriate.

I was awoken just after noon by the shrill voice of Mom calling out my name. I had to get up and get into the kitchen so we could talk. I was hoping Dad would be awake, but he had finally fallen asleep, and once asleep, there was no waking him up.

I took the seat across from Mom at the kitchen table, and she started with her speech. She would tell me she was discussing school, but she was really telling me how it was going to be. I sat in silence as she went through how God wanted me to do something with my life other than write stories about demons and vampires or directing movies filled with all sorts of monsters.

When she finally finished, I told her I was unconcerned about what her God wanted me to do. How could she even know what God wanted? If He was talking to her, He needed to stop by the house when I was home and talk with me. But like every other time, God was a no show. If He could not show up, how could I ever know what He wanted, and why would He tell my mother?

With her pleas for God falling on dead ears, she made an offer. If I went to Liberty University, she would pay for the entire four years, plus living expenses. I just had to go. For some reason she did not seem to hear what I was saying. If I was not going to play my education around God, why would I ever go to Liberty University—a Christian school ran by Jerry Falwell and his right wing followers? I would rather just go to work and not even go to school than to set foot on Liberty's campus.

She continued to talk, but I just kept telling her no. I had figured out a way to get to film school without her assistance. Dad would always be there to help out if I found myself in a tight spot. I had tuition and living expenses taken care of; I just needed to get to Orlando by September.

Her arguments were not enough to change my mind, but she did something I never expected. She pulled off her wig and started to cry at the table. I was sitting across from my mother as she pleaded with me to stay. It was a low blow, but it worked. I could not stomach to see my mother crying to just keep me around. She looked so sick and frail.

I told her I would go to Ohio State in the fall instead of film school. I would do a couple of years there until David graduated from high school and then transfer to Orlando. I would not leave her. I would stay just to prevent the sobs. I was torn between two loves, that of film and that of my family. If I left, I would be leaving David to tend to Mom on his own; if I stayed I would be giving up the opportunity of a lifetime.

With OSU as the college choice, Mom could now brag to her friends at church about what I was doing. Before, she had been ashamed of everything I was doing other than getting good grades in school. She never talked about the dance competitions I won, or the theater productions I was involved in, or the stories I was writing, but now she had something other than great academics to boast about.

I was not sure want I would be studying now, but I knew I would be involved in the theater department and take everything I could in Cinematography. Mom would have everyone think I would come around once I got into school and do something a little more prestigious such as political science, law, or medicine. She always seemed to want for me the exact opposite of what I wanted. I am not sure if it was my teenage desire to find my place or that my mother and I were two very different people seeking very different things in life, but we never seemed to see the same future.

38

The End of Childhood

With the high school graduation ceremony behind me, the rest of my life was just beginning. Everything that had come before would be a stepping stone to what lay ahead. Before stepping out into the world, I took one final trip to New York with the local theater group. When I returned to Ohio, the fun carefree times of the weeks and years filled with high school, dances, and long nights playing video games would be over. Life with work, financial responsibility, and nights filled with cramming for college classes now lay ahead.

Supporting myself in college would take more than a job at a local theater. It was time for me to take a job, not because it was something I wanted, but something that would pay the electric and allow me to eat. Mom would still be around to help, but I had to start to take on some of the monetary responsibilities. Mom was paying for college, the least I could do was feed and cloth myself, pay for my own insurance, etc.

With Mom's connections and good standing at Nationwide, she was able to secure me a job at the Nationwide claims center in Worthington. The pay was far better than anything I would have found on my own, and the hours were set up around my school schedule during the day. I only had to deal with working, not only for the same company as my mother, but in the same building, on the same floor. She would be just across the hall.

It would seem no matter how hard I tried to get away—to not be reminded of her condition, I would not be able to separate myself from her. During the weeks and months when her treatments were going well, she would be at work, often getting ready to leave as I was pulling in to start my shift. It seemed she knew everyone in the company. Everyone I spoke with wanted to know how she was doing if she had not come in, and it always felt like I was being watched. Mom's little spies were everywhere when I went to work.

This first job would be the beginning of a trap that would later suffocate me in the monotonous routine and unfilled vision of what could and should have been.

In high school, I had been working for the fun of work and what that effort entailed. Going into college, I was working out of necessity. Work no longer was fun, it had become work. It had become something that had to be done in order to achieve other goals and maintain a standard of living.

Not only had my job changed, but my friends had changed as well. All through high school I had been told to say goodbye to everyone at graduation. The likelihood of ever seeing any of the childhood friends after that final day of school would be slim. Each of us would go in many different directions and our paths would most likely never cross again in our lives.

Just two months after high school was out, everyone I knew seemed to be distant memories. Occasionally, I would see someone from school as I drove through Centerburg or Mount Vernon, but other than that random encounter, they were all gone. It was like they had never existed.

The bonds that had taken years to develop were dissolved in a matter of weeks. It makes me wonder if any of us were actually friends to begin with or just close associates held together by the common threat of high school. When that thread was finally cut, everyone went their own way, wishing them the best, but deeply grateful they would no longer be forced to be nice to people they never really liked.

A new job, new friends—it was only time before new goals began to seep into my life. For years, I had worked towards graduating from high school. Now I was working towards something new. Film school was still in my sights, and I never let go of the dream of going, but I had to realize that it may be a long way off and that doing well at Ohio State was the most paramount of my concerns now.

Before my goals had been developed around the dreams I had had as a boy, now they were wrapped around my survival in the world. I had to ensure I would be able to pay the obligations life through at me and my concern had to stay focused on this new agenda. Self supportiveness was the first goal that would hopefully give me something to stand on as I continued to reach for the director chair and the published novel.

No longer was I a kid in a world outlined by teachers and my parents. I was an adult in a chaotic world that I would need to make sense of in order to find direction. The next few years would be spent looking for the points of the compass and moving in a consistent direction that would make me a productive part of the new world around me. The maps of my high school years were no longer valid. I would have to find my own way without the safety of past friends, past guidance, or past experiences.

Everything was new; everything was dangerous. There were so many roads that would lead to the rest of my life. Choosing the right one would be the test that would only be graded when I looked back after many years of living with the outcome of my choices.

39

College

It had finally come. The moment I had been looking forward to since starting high school. I was out on my own without the constant supervision of Mom. I moved into my dorm just a week before the start of the fall semester and could not wait to get started. Even though I was not at the school of my choice or studying that which was most passionate to me, I still could not wait for the first day of class.

Just like with my senior year at Mount Vernon High School, I would start the school year off with Mom going into the hospital for a new treatment for her cancer. The extensive chemotherapy and painful radiation treatments had failed to put the tumors in her body into remission. The only hope she had left at life was a bone marrow transplant.

Just as I was moving into the dorm room that would be my home for the next year, Mom was entering the James Cancer Institute on the Ohio State campus. For the next month she would be locked in a room, completely separated from anyone other than the doctors and the nurses in charge of her care. Everyday after class I would go to her room and look in on her through the glass windows.

Sometimes she would be able to talk with me, other days she would only be able to look over, too wore out to talk. As others came to visit, they would leave her cards of support or little trinkets to brighten her day. She was not able to have much in her room, so would I gather the presents and put them in my car before going to work. I would take them to the house on one of my many visits to check up on David and make sure Dad was not driving everyone crazy.

After she had been released from the hospital and on her way to recovering from the transplant, my mind was at greater ease, and I was able to really start enjoying my first year of college life. For the last two years, I had worried about the treatments she was undergoing, but for once they were all over. There was nothing left to try in her fight with cancer. The only thing left was to endure was time. Time would let us all know if the radical treatment worked, but the nights filled with sickness and pain were over for her. Hope was all that was left.

Dorm living quickly became some of the best times in my life. Being in a coed dorm, the ladies on one floor and the men on the other, and no matter what time of the day it was, there was always someone to hang with and something to do. Many nights were filled with shaving cream wars, lots of loud music, and food everywhere you looked.

I had brought the typewriter Dad had bought me years before, but soon found I would need something more to get through all the papers I would be writing and to help with research. It was time for me to move up to a complete computer system. The old typewriter with its ink ribbons and pin wheel served its purpose in high school and allowed me to explore many of my stories of terror, but it had become inadequate.

Just two weeks into school I bought my first computer. It was top of the line with Windows 3.1, a 166 MHz Pentium processor, a 14.4 internal fax modem, and a full gigabyte on its hard drive. It even came with a voucher to get the new Windows 95 when it released later that month.

When I got it back to my room and hooked it up, it was the most power computer in the dorm. I signed up for America Online and began to surf a web with very little out there to look at, but even with the few websites, instant messaging was really cool and the e-mail function looked like it would be something I would be able to use.

This first computer would be the beginning of an obsession to have the best and most powerful. I would spend thousands of dollars playing with the newest and best computer technology. Some guys had cars. They would do everything they could to get a little more horsepower out of their engines. I had computers; always looking for more storage and faster processing speed.

With the winning streak of the Buckeyes, weekend partying made going to class bearable. I was always looking forward to Friday, especially when Saturday's game would be at the Horse Shoe. A home game meant the clubs would be filled with the ladies and beer would be flowing in fountains.

On game night, it seemed like everyone in Columbus rushed to the Main Street clubs to party along with the winning team. The sidewalks would be so packed, people spilt out onto the streets with their beers in hand. Traffic would come to a stand still as the police struggled to keep the students in the clubs, frat houses, or anywhere but the street. Eventually they would give up and simply just try to keep the rowdy crowds from doing too much property damage or fights from getting too far out of hand.

On those nights, I would go out with friends, from club to club, house to house, drinking all the free booze I could get and meeting new people to party with on the next game night. I managed to make it back to my dorm each night, but after the Notre Dame victory I was picked up after walking into a street sign. The police eventually let me go after they had detained so many students there was not enough room for everyone. The cops just started writing tickets to everyone and sending us on our merry way.

The nights filled with celebration in football mite was only heightened by Sorority Rush, something I had not heard of until I started seeing woman everywhere doing all kinds of wild stunts to pledge their preferred sorority. I would spend many hours in the Oval tossing a football waiting for the topless girls to streak through. I was able to see more naked woman on the campus lawn that year than I would see in all my nights at the clubs or at private parties.

I was having a great time, but the fun times came to quick halt as the end of the first term sneaked up on me. I was spending so much time out with the ladies, out at the bars, or hitting the frat house parties, my classes had become second to my night life. With weak grades throughout the semester, the only chances I had left were finals. Finals were my last possibility of making the passing grades needed to move forward into the winter semester.

I spent my Thanksgiving break knee deep in books making up for lost time. I had two weeks to cram three months worth of studies in order to pass. I was surprised when I got back to the dorms after the short break to see everyone was doing the same thing I was doing. The entire dorm seemed to shut down as we all struggled to compress the knowledge of a semester into two weeks of study.

No longer were the lounges filled with people playing pool or video games, they were filled with stacks of books and near silence. Each of us would help others in subjects we excelled in for the return service in subjects we struggled in. The months of binge drinking had caught up with us, but we all pulled together to get everyone through the next two weeks. We all wanted to stay, and we needed each other to pull it off.

I just barely made it. I passed all my finals with high enough grades to pass the classes. I would be returning after winter break along with everyone in the dorm. With all of us working together, not a one of the eighty or so students who had partied their nights away had failed their classes. Most of us had learned our lessons and would be truly starting college after Christmas. The first semester was just for us to get to know one another and have fun doing it.

The wild times were out of my system; only in moderation would I be hitting the bars or spending all night out with friends. I had barely missed a catastrophe and did not want to have to endure another two weeks like those before finals.

Unlike the fall semester, I registered for winter classes. Mom had selected courses for me to take during the fall because I did not want to go to Ohio State and figured I would be able to get out of going if I did not sign up for the classes. I figured film school would be the only option left for me to do during the fall if I just let the OSU registration deadlines pass without a response. But my inaction did not work with her. She took care of everything for the fall, but I made a point to handle the winter registration.

I am not sure what my mother was thinking about when she filled out the paperwork for my courses. I ended up taking Chemistry, Biology, Calculus, and Advance English. She loaded me up with some of the hardest classes a freshman could take, and none of them, for the exception of the English, were anything I had any interest in. Even if I had not spent my time partying hard, it would have been tough for me to get grades much higher then what I actually ended up with after a hard cram session.

When I finally was able to talk to my academic advisor, I found out I was pre-med, something as far from cinematography as a student could get. I changed my major to one of communications and enrolled in two theater classes, a literature class, and a computer class, making sure these classes would roll over to film school—no sense wasting my time at Ohio State. I was not where I wanted to be, but at least I would gain something that would help when I did get where I wanted to go.

With the new semester starting, I was able to get back into the theater. I had had to drop my job at the theater in Mount Vernon in order to take the one at Nationwide, and I was unable to be a part of the Mount Vernon Players due to my schedule, but the theater classes put me back on the stage, and this time I was getting college credit.

During my first production for the theater class, a problem came up that had been with me at the dorm and back in high school. I had over looked it twice but this third time was enough; it had become a nuisance that just would not go away. Another student in the class had the same name as me. There was another Christopher Harris working on the same production with me. There was a different Christopher Harris living two floors above me in my dorm, and at Centerburg High School there was yet another Christopher Harris. It is rare for most of us to me someone with the same first and last name during our entire lives, but I had met three in just a thirty mile radius.

In high school, I had been separated from the other Chris Harris by our middle initials. In the dorm we were separated by numbers. I was Chris One the other was Chris Three due to the floors we were living on. In theater class, we were separated by the name of the characters we played. I became known as Trent, and he became known as Jason.

There were two other people from my floor working on the production with me, and it did not take long for the entire dorm to be referring to me as Trent instead of Chris One. The new name even made it to Nationwide. It became a nickname that stuck, making the name Christopher simply the name that was on official papers, but I was known to everyone as Trent.

The new name drew a clear line between the new and the old. I could easily tell who was calling on the phone or who was looking for me by the name they used. No one but those from Centerburg or from Lynchburg knew me as Christopher. All of the new people I came in contact with knew me as Trent. If someone referred to me as Christopher, they were pre-college associates; everyone asking for Trent was a new friend or co-worker.

When the police came to the dorm looking for Christopher Harris, the problem that just seemed to be a statistical anomaly became an issue of mistaken identity. The RA came and got me and Chris Three and brought us to the lounge on the request of an arresting officer. It was later discovered they were not looking for either of us but yet another Chris Harris on the campus. It seemed he was wanted for eluding police and for selling counterfeit basketball tickets.

In class the next day I had found out the Chris Harris known as Jason was also harassed by the police because of the deeds of someone else with our name. A pre-law student overheard our complaining and suggested we change our names. He even offered to help out if we allowed him to use us as project on legal procedure for one of his other classes.

He did not have to convince me; I had lived with being mistaken for another Chris for the better part of four years. By February of 1996, Christopher Lee Harris became Trenton Michael Harris. The change over in college and at work went very smoothly, everyone already knew me as Trent. It would take some time for those back in Centerburg to get used to the new name, but in just a few years everyone in Centerburg would know the name Trent M. Harris.

As the school year began to wind down, I was doing much better academically. I was back into the theater. The job at Nationwide was going well, and I had a new name. The only thing left was my own place. I was not looking forward to going home for the summer to live. I had been bitten by the bug of independence and did not want to go back under the thumb of Mom. I was also sure

I did not want to live in a dorm the next year. It was fun while it lasted, but I needed a place of my own.

Just as finals were over and the summer break began, I moved into my first apartment just off Lane Avenue overlooking the Horse Shoe and St John Arena. Instead of taking my stuff home, I just moved it from my dorm to my new place. It was not the best place—just a studio apartment, but several of my friends lived in the building. I could hang out with them when I wanted, then go back to my place when I needed some quiet time. In the dorm, quiet time was a sought after luxury, but here I would have it anytime I wanted.

During the summer, I spent my days working with a Columbus theatrical group and worked at Nationwide in the evenings. I took several trips to the beach and Lake Erie with friends, but in general it was a quiet summer. I remained in contact with the film school and the studio in Florida in the hopes of transferring after just one more year at Ohio State. I scheduled classes for the next year I was certain would transfer over. Repeating classes was something I wanted to avoid at all costs. Repeating would be a waste of time.

During my summer down time, I began to write again. It had been almost a year since I had written anything creative. Not going to the school of my choice and dealing with Mom's illness had drained some of the creative juices I once had overflowing when I wrote *A Murder Story* and *Awakening*.

It was time to get back to telling the horror stories I so loved as a boy. That summer the first draft of *Christopher* was written on the computer bought to write term papers and to do research for classes. For the exception of a few short stories, I had not published anything since *A Murder Story*, but the act of just writing something new kept the dreams and hopes of one day seeing my work in print alive. As the new story began to develop and the pages began to build, the desire to go to film school was re-ignited with a fire that would make it hard to wait just one more year.

In just one more year, I would be in Florida looking out my apartment window at Palm trees and sand instead of Oaks and concrete. The knee deep snow of Ohio's winters would be something of the past, replaced by Christmas in shorts and t-shirts. Instead of going to class with my eyes on something else, I would finally be were I wanted to be. I would finally be learning the skills to develop that which I loved most.

I started the next fall at Ohio State, keeping my eye on May. That would be the month I could leave. That would be the month when I could finally follow a dream I had had for as long as I could remember. May would be the month of passage from dreams to reality.

40

The End Closes In

Just a few weeks into my sophomore year at OSU, the tests came back for Mom. After a year of waiting, we would finally know whether the bone marrow transplant had worked. We would finally know if the battles had won the war or simply postponed the inevitable.

I took the day off from work and hurried home right after class. Again, Mary had gone with Mom to the oncologist, and both were home when I pulled into the driveway early that afternoon. In a reversing role, I was the one walking through the living room door; they were the ones waiting.

Unlike when they had come home to tell David and I Mom had cancer, I was riding on the cloud of hope. I just knew the bone marrow treatment had worked. Anything that aggressive had to at least stop the tumors from spreading if not putting them into remission. Mom had fought for so long and extended her life through chemotherapy treatments and radiation treatments, this would be no different.

I was desperately hoping for complete remission, but I would accept just an extension with the anticipation of a better cure. She had extended her life from six months when she was first diagnosed with cancer to almost two years. She had done this through sheer will and desire to live. All of that energy fighting would finally pay off.

I threw my coat on the sofa and went into the kitchen where Mary and Mom were sitting at the table. Just as I stepped across the threshold, the hopes I had coming into the house evaporated. Both of the ladies were crying over the coffee they were trying to sip down. I did not need to be told, the sense in the room spoke loud enough.

The cancer was not in remission. It had not stopped growing. Instead, it was on the move throughout her body. There was nothing anyone could do to stop its spread. Everything she had done to fight had only been for two years filled with many nights of tremendous pain, nausea, hair loss, and the inability to do the things she once held in high regard. She gave up her last good times in life to struggle in a loosing mêlée.

I sat down and waited for Mom to gather herself enough to tell me the cancer was growing out of control. She explained the circumstances the way the doctors had, using complicated blood counts and other medical jargon, but I had all I needed. I just needed to know what she was going to do next. She seemed to always have the next step planned out, and I was ready to support her in whatever decision she made.

For the first time in my life, Mom did not have an answer. Her next move was to do nothing but pray and enjoy whatever life she had left to live. Undergoing more chemotherapy and radiation would extend her life, but the quality of that life would not be worth living. She did not want to endure anymore more nights crippled by illness. She did not want to have to stay away from her friends and family while her immune system rebuilt itself after treatments. She no longer wanted to eat only those foods best for her heath. She no longer wanted to miss church and the fellowship of serving God because of illness.

Her life was not over in her mind—just limited. She knew the end would be here sooner than she would have liked, but she was determined to look ahead and press forward. Whatever life she had left would be spent living life. Mom had lived for forty some years, but the last few months of her life would be her best and would impact the people around her in ways she could not fully comprehend and in ways I am just beginning to understand.

As I watched her and spent time with her those last few months, I wondered what kind of a life a person could build for themselves if they knew the next few months would be their last. We seem to get more things done when we know the deadline or have a good idea when time is running out. Life seems to radiate from us when death is just around the corner.

Mom choose these last few months to extend her hand to everyone she could reach. She choose to help those around her in anyway she could. Her help would be the lasting impression people would have when she was gone. They would remember her for the step up she gave them when they needed it the most.

While she was helping out those around her, she expressed her first interest in the things I thought were important. She never liked the theater, the drill teams, or writing while in high school, but she did attend a college play and came to several of my drill competitions. For the first time in my life, I had a family member in the audience while I was on stage. I had a parent cheering me on as my drill team stomped the competition with our fast paced dance moves timed with perfect acrobatic chorography.

I do not think she ever approved of the goals I sought to achieve, but she wanted to know and to see her son in his own environment before she passed away. For once, my life was not about what she wanted for it, but what I wanted. It felt good to have her in the audience, and I was proud to introduce her to everyone as my mother.

As the holidays approached, David and I knew this would most likely be the last Thanksgiving and Christmas we would have with her. We did everything we could to make these two holidays the best we could not only for her but for ourselves as well. These would be the freshest memories of our mother after her passing, and we wanted them to be good ones.

Anything she wanted she got. If she wanted to go Christmas caroling with her church group, we made sure she did. If she wanted David and I in church for Thanksgiving and Christmas service, we were there. I even said the blessing for the dinners—something I had never done, even though she had asked many times.

Time, which seemed in abundance all my life, was now in short supply. Every minute needed to be the best it could be—second chances would not be given this time around. There would not be other Christmas celebrations or dinners. These were the last for her, and the last I would have with her.

The private dinners and talks that had started after Mom first found out she had cancer changed those last few months. Before we would talk about school, working things out with Dad, looking out for David, but they turned into the final farewells discussions. She made sure I knew that she loved me and apologized for what she perceived to be mistakes in her past.

I had once looked forward to having our modest mother-son dinners. In college I had little money, and the food I could buy was not always the best. A nice steak dinner was always welcome, even if it was with my mother instead of my girlfriend and college buds. Over those meals, she had told me about the family. She let me know where I had come from and what part my distant family in Virginia had played in her life and in mine.

Now I tried to avoid these intimate conversations. I did not want her to tell me goodbye, or tell apologize for things I never thought were problems until she brought them up. I did not want to tell her goodbye. I was not ready for what lay ahead, and this kind of talk just seemed to expedite the unavoidable.

Other than those few times when she talked about leaving, the cancer had been forgotten. For a couple of months, everything seemed to be normal. Mom had put back on the weight she had lost during her treatments and her hair had grown back in. She was not exactly the same as she was just two years earlier, but for once in a long time the disease she had was not written all over her, through her gaunt eyes, smooth head, and skinny frame. If you did not know, one would think she was in perfect health.

When Christmas was over, I registered for my winter semester, and David got ready to return to school. We had been given the gift of a couple of months with her, but almost immediately after the New Year, mom started to deteriorate. When classes finally started, she was already on morphine, with everything being done now only to alleviate the pain, to make the passing comfortable.

For the first couple of weeks, David would help her with her morphine each night before going to bed. Mom disliked having anyone take care of her other than those she knew as family or very close friends. For a while, David became her care giver. I would come in when I could each week, but the weights had been placed on his shoulders.

Eventually Dad came up for a while to help out as best he could. Trying to help a dying ex-wife was not an easy task, but he knew David could not be left there alone as his mother slowly succumbed. During this time, the battle of wills between and David and Dad started to develop as each thought they had a better way of doing things around the house. I would often have to be the referee between the two to keep the fists from swinging or the language from getting too far out of hand.

These fights between the two would be something that would last for the rest of my Dad's life. No matter what anyone did, David and Dad would be at each others throats—constantly instigating fights to get back at one another for the lost fights of the past. There were two men living in a house that could not get along; I was living in Columbus, and the household was falling apart. Household activities were being done from a totally male perspective. The house was quickly turning into a bachelor pad with dirty dishes lining the kitchen counters, vacuuming became a thing of the past, and God help anyone who went into the bathroom.

It was evident Mom was the cornerstone to my home. She had been the one who kept everything running in an efficient manner. With her ex-husband and two sons at the wheel, a totally new set of standards had crept in and were taking over one room at a time.

Hospice was finally brought in to guide Dad and David, to ensure everything was getting done as it should in the manner it should. They were invited in as Mom went from going out to talk with her friends to being able to just call them on the phone. Her time spent out with the people she loved was over. Our house became the entire world. The outside was no longer acceptable.

Coming home on frequent visits, I saw Mom loose the weight she had gained, a sunken look crept back in around her eyes, and her skin slowly started to turn yellow and pasty. I watcher her go from a woman able to go outside, to have dinners with friends at her favorite restaurants, to a woman home bond and then later bedridden as the cancer seemed to speed up its attack on her body.

Within just a few weeks, Mom became a lump in a bed, unable to sit up, unable to talk, unable to do anything but look out into the room, looking for the end. Everything I knew of her was gone—replaced by a shell that at times did not even know who I was. Before her body ever gave up on life, she was gone. She was still living, but I would never be able to talk to her again. I would never have to eat the food she called dinner again. I no longer had the opportunity to tell her the things I wanted to say before she died. The time was up. I was just waiting for her body to catch up with her mind and soul.

41

She Left

Hospice had been in and out of the house for several weeks, but Brenda had taken charge of caring for my mother as she struggled for her last moments of life. Mom was very particular as to who she wanted caring for her at a time when she would be the weakest. She did not like strangers in her house. When Wanda was unable to be there and David and I were unable to do the things needed to care for her, Brenda came in and filled the gaps.

Ever since I could remember, Brenda and her family had been a part of my life. Her oldest son, Jason, has been a friend of mine since grade school. Mom was repeatedly taking me over to his house for sleepovers or to work on school projects. Later Brenda would take her family to the church I attended and, from there, a friendship developed between her and Mom. They had been social before meeting in church, but their time together worshipping God really solidified their closeness.

When Brenda first came in to help out with Mom, I finally was able to relax a little. Before there had been strangers in my home caring for her. Wanda was there for a portion of the time to help out, but there was nothing like having Brenda in the house. She knew me personally and knew my history. She had a part in my past, and that part gave me a sense of easiness that few people were able to provide. With her, it was like an old friend visiting at a time when I needed it the most.

In a span of a month, my mother had went from sleeping in her bed, still resembling the woman I once knew, to a woman in a hospital bed in the backroom, her skin and eyes beginning to yellow as her liver succumbed to the ravages of the cancer. On her dresser, she had rows of pill bottles to help with the symptoms of the cancer treatments, but they were all collecting dust as they were useless now. The only bottle used was the one containing morphine. Treating the disease was now just a failed hope. The only treatable symptom left was the pain.

The pain was the only thing left our sciences could stave off as disease ran uncontrollably through her body.

During the week of March 24, 1997, I had taken much of the week off from work. Mom was unable to get out of her bed, and David was in school. Dad and I were the ones left to take care of the house the best we could with the hordes of people traipsing through saying their final goodbyes to my mother. My supervisors at Nationwide eventually moved my work hours later into the evening, giving me time to get everything in order at home during the day and work at night.

On March 24th, 1997, I went and said goodbye to Mom and headed for Columbus to pull my shift at work. I had been absent for several days and needed to get out of the house for a little bit, even if it was to go to work. When I told her goodbye, I kissed on her forehead and squeezed her hand. I am positive she knew who I was even though just hours before she had not even been able to talk or sit up. As I walked out of her room, I blotted out her sunken checks, her lemon yellow eyes, and the smell of death that lingered in her room and replaced it with an image of her in my past, long before cancer visited my home.

I got to work around six that evening, David had gone out with his friends and Dad would be at the house with Brenda for the night. I was unable to receive calls at work but gave Dad and Brenda my pager number and told them to beep me if they needed anything. I would be able to call them as soon as possible and pick up anything they needed on my way home.

After just an hour of work, I did get a page from home. I never expected a call from home unless something was wrong with Mom. Dad and Brenda were able to handle anything that would come up. As the pager vibrated in my pocket, I excused myself from work and went to the break room to make a call. I could have made the call from my desk, but I knew the news I was going to get and wanted to be alone. I wanted to be away from the people as I heard the news my mother had died.

From a payphone, Brenda told me Mom had died, and I needed to come home as soon as possible. I was the first called and needed to find David before going home. On the hour long drive home, I called Marilyn and asked if she could find David for me. Even though she had not directly cared for David and I for several years, she still kept up with the two of us and was the one I knew would be able to track my brother down.

It did not take but a few moments to hear back from Marilynn on car phone that she had found David and that he was waiting at her house. I am not sure if David knew Mom had passed away or simply thought Marilyn wanted to see him, but I stopped by before going home and told my brother our mother had died.

Telling David that Mom had died while he waited in Marilynn's living room was not as hard as returning home that night. David and I both knew for a good while that at any moment we would get the news she had left us, but returning home that night was worse then getting the news.

When I pulled into the driveway, the light in my mother's room was on, and I knew she was in that room in her bed and no longer living. Earlier that night I had left my home with a complete family. Just a few hours later, I was returning to a broken family with no hopes of ever putting it back together. With David following my lead we went in. Brenda was in the kitchen and Dad was back in the room with Mom.

It was finally over for the David and I. No longer would we have to sleep in a house filled with moans of pains and tears of fear. We would not longer have to go the hospitals and watch as the radiation burned our Mom. No longer would our hopes be lifted by some new drug or treatment only to be crushed with the realities of the disease. No longer would we have to watch our mother suffer as she fought for just one more day of life.

With her death, Mom was released from her torments, and David and I had been freed from uncertainty and the crushing weight of death. We could now deal with the loss of our mother and move on instead of waiting on the inevitable.

That night David, Dad, and I said goodbye one final time before the funeral home came to take her body away. Each of us had our own way of dealing with what had happened. David immersed himself in videogames; Dad had a bottle of Vodka, and I dove into the newest Stephen King terror. None of us really slept that night. After the phone calls to the family, we had nothing to do but wait. It was too late to start the funeral process. We were just left with our thoughts and a quiet house.

The next morning the three of us left, woke up early from a night with very little sleep and started a new day without the woman who had built our life in Ohio, who had been the one to provide everything for David and I throughout our lives. With all of us up and moving, it did not take long before we all wanted to leave. The house was closing in on us. Everywhere we looked we saw remnants of her and her illness.

David was the first to leave, followed by Dad and I. Mom's friend Mary had come by early with some Egg McMuffins, and we left her in charge of the house. With a note affixed to the door letting everyone know to call Mary for the funeral arrangements, we left. We went wherever we could to get away. The funeral had already been taken care of by Mom long before she became very ill; we just had to show up. With that already handled, Dad and I only needed to go shopping for some news cloths for the funeral. I already had several suits, but he did not, and David needed a new jacket.

The day after her death was spent dealing with her loss in private, just between the family. That evening and next few days would be filled with talking to friends and extended family, but this time was ours. By the time our day of private mourning was over, Mom's sisters had shown up and family friends were starting to filter in with dishes of home cooked food.

I never really understood why people want to come to the home of a person who has died unless they are immediate family. The deceased person is no longer there. More than likely, the families of the deceased are usually strangers to them, but they still come over. I always thought that was what the viewing and funeral service was for, but they came in droves and trampled through my house at a time when I just needed some quiet.

As the funeral approached, mourners eventually stopped popping in, saving their remarks of condolences for the service. It was not that I did not want to see the people, I just needed a place to go to be alone, and they were taking it away from me by constantly filling my living room and kitchen. I was looking forward for a few days with just the closest friends and family. I was looking forward to just watching a movie, soaking in what had happened, without having to entertain someone or a group of people.

When it was time for the viewing, we were asked to be at the funeral home an hour before the start so we could make sure everything was the way Mom wanted and to take care of any last minute preparations. The last time I had seen my mother was the night she had died. She was in her bed unable to muster the strength to sit up or tell me goodbye as I left for work. This time she would be in her casket. The image of her lifeless in her bed did not seem as final as seeing her lying in her casket. In her bed there was the illusion of hope; in the casket everything was final.

Mom's sisters were able to say goodbye before the first visitors had arrived, and David and I were given the events that would occur on that night and how the funeral would be conducted the next day.

By the time the night was over, I had shaken many hands, accepted many condolences and was ready for the evening to end. The faces of the people started to blur at one point, and the last couple of hours were spent out back smoking, avoiding the sympathies of those inside the funeral home.

The viewing was for those who had not seen Mom in a while or who were not able to be with her the last few days of her life to tell her goodbye. I just assumed to wait outside while they talked about the past, about special moments in their lives that included the company of my mother. Many of them were strangers to me; I was only known through the vicarious conversations Mom had had with them at work or at church.

Before moving out back to smoke and spend time with my friends, I noticed the very distinctive groups who had shown up. Each group had a different way of describing my mother's life. They each saw her through different eyes and different circumstances. The visitors from church saw her as a Godly woman, those from Nationwide saw her as a hard worker, David and I saw her as a mother, her family from Virginia remembered her as a child, and her friends talked about the good times they had had, but no one seemed to have a complete picture.

The full picture lay in the many people that were there that night to send her off. As individuals, only a part of Mom's life was represented. As a group I could see the entire woman she had grown to be and the life she had lived. I could finally see her for the person she was and how she had interacted and changed the world around her.

The next day, everyone who meant anything to her and to David and I gathered for the funeral and said our final farewells. The day was bright and had a spring like feel to it as David and I said goodbye to her and began the first steps into a world without the overbearing protection of a loving mother.

While walking back to our cars, Mom's good friend Mary came up to me and gave me a booklet of stories written by the people Mom had worked with at Nationwide. I read those stories that night, and in every word written, I saw my mother and her dedication to providing for her two sons. The experiences these coworkers had with her were a part of her life I was not privy to growing up. I just knew she worked in insurance but had little contact with the life she lived while at work.

I have included these stories because they represent a part of her life I am not about to describe other than say she far exceeded the expectations of many people when she first made the move to Ohio to take a job. This is what her Nationwide family had to say about her.

In October of November of 1981, just after we had moved to Columbus (Charlotte from Lynchburg, me from Syracuse), we decided to take a drive in my brand new Chevy Citation down to Bob Evans Farms, about an hour south of Columbus.

It was a beautiful day, crisp and clear. Charlotte and I and her two boys, Christopher and David, who must have been about five and three years old at the time, had breakfast at a Bob Evans restaurant. Our server gave the boys crayons so they could draw and color on their placemats.

After breakfast, we piled back into the car and headed toward Bob Evans Farms. Charlotte and I were talking and the boys were being quiet in the back when David suddenly piped up, "Mama, isn't this pretty?" He had drawn a picture with his new crayons on the back of my new front seat.

Charlotte very calmly told me, "When you get a moment, please pull the car over."

"Why?" I asked, wondering if one of the boys was sick. I didn't know about the work of art.

As soon as I could, I pulled over into a parking lot belonging to a church. Charlotte got out of the car, opened the back door for David, pulled him out, and proceeded to wale the tar out of his little behind—in the church parking lot!

When Charlotte and David were finished with their business, they got back into the car, and we drove on to Bob Evans Farms.

Kathy

◆   ◆   ◆

Look up the word "inspiration" in the dictionary, and you will see a picture of Charlotte.

Ray

◆   ◆   ◆

I have only known Charlotte for about two years. She has been a great inspiration for me. The times that I would call to inquire how she was doing and to offer encouragement, the call always ended with her making me feel good.

I have never met a more caring and inspirational person as Charlotte. May God bless!

Nancy

◆   ◆   ◆

Charlotte's neighbor was my second cousin. When he passed away of cancer, she was there for me. I hope to be there for her. I have worked with her for years; we were very close.

Charlotte taught me to be a stronger person. I have met many people in this life, and she is one I will never forget. We are only three months apart in age, but I always let her know she was older than me during those three months. Charlotte and I have a lot in common: she has two sons and so do I. They are about the same ages. She is a strong person.

I will never forget when she came to National Accounts and told us the story of how she got her job at Nationwide. Her father was working at a bank, and she helped him. Nationwide hired her in the accounting department. They thought she had some experience working at the bank, not knowing she knew nothing about accounting or working for a bank. Her father was a janitor at the bank, and she helped him there. She couldn't even use a calculator! When she was told to add a stack of drafts, Charlotte got a notepad and pencil and started adding the drafts on paper!

Toni

◆   ◆   ◆

From working at Nationwide for many years, I had known Charlotte only as a fellow employee I had seen around the office.

That changed in January 1991, when I took a new position as the systems manager in our Office of National Accounts. My responsibilities were to support the computer systems needs of the other area of the office, which included Charlotte's area.

My first memory of any work contact with Charlotte was in a manager's meeting I attended shortly after assuming my new job. As the newest member of this team of about 12 managers, I remember being very concerned about getting off to a good start with my new peers. In this meeting I made a comment, which, at the time, I thought was rather non-controversial. Charlotte took exception and responded as such in a rather strong manner. I felt somewhat under attack and remembered thinking I had two options: (1) get into a debate with a peer I did not know in front of all my other peers; or (2) handle outside the meeting. I wisely chose the latter.

At that point, I must admit, I had serious thoughts as to what type of working relationship we would have. Little did I know that it was the beginning of what would become a great friendship.

Over the next two-and-a-half years, Charlotte and I worked as a team on numerous projects and came to respect one another as professionals.

More importantly, we came to know one another as fellow Christians and personal friends. We spent time talking about our faith in God and His promise of everlasting life through our Savior Jesus Christ. We spoke of our families and our dreams. Charlotte was always telling me stories about what her sons were doing. They were the pride and joy of her life. We worked together on the difficult task of closing our office in 1993.

Over the past two-and-a-half years, since Charlotte was diagnosed with cancer, we spoke on many occasions about her health, the treatments, and her sons. Most of all, Charlotte would always talk about her love of and her faith in God. Never once did she ever show the slightest hint of any doubts in His power over her life. She knew that God could heal her and was prepared to accept whatever His will was.

Her faith was always inspiring to me. Sometimes when we would talk, I might be dealing with something that was bothering me, and after a few minutes of conversation with Charlotte, I would feel encouraged by her strong faith. She would always have a scripture to recite of that she wanted me to read.

When I think of Charlotte, I don't think of the positions she held or the influential people she knew and worked with. I will always remember her as a devoted mother and woman of unbending faith in her God.

Richard

◆   ◆   ◆

Charlotte made an impact on my life by standing by us when National Accounts decentralized. She encouraged us to bring our resumes to her so she could read them over and advise us on improving them. She also read verses form Psalms to give us spiritual strength. She also let us see the vulnerable side of her while she underwent treatment for cancer and her never ending strength and faith throughout.

I respect and admire her for her strong faith and courage and will never forget her.

Rosemary

◆   ◆   ◆

In 1977, I was transferred to Virginia as the Customer Services division manager. In those days, we didn't have offices, just filing cabinets around us.

On my second day on the job, Charlotte presented herself in front of my desk and said, "Mr. Dusenbury, my name is Charlotte Harris," in her finest southern belle drawl. "I am the mail room supervisor, and I am her to explain how we address mail in VARO." With that, she handed me a few things that I had mailed wrong!

From that day on, I have been a devout fan of Charlotte's and have had three or four professional duties where she touched my life and our customers.

Christopher and David, I want to tell you how much I love your mama and how very privileged I have been to work with her. Her patience and invincible enthusiasm for doing the right thing and doing things right will be her unflinching legacy in my mind.

Francis

◆   ◆   ◆

I remember when Charlotte first bought her house. The land was flat and bare because it was farmland. She bought 100 pine seedlings from the forest service or some other government agency and planted them. One hundred seedlings is a lot of plant-ing—they were less than a foot high.

I remember grousing about the day lilies in my yard, how they were taking over, and that I was going to have to pull them out like weeds. Charlotte said that's what she needed, so I dug them out and gave them to her. She planted them in her front yard, near the ditch.

I haven't been out the house since them, but I imagine it now, not as a farmer's field, but as a standard suburban home with trees and shrubs and wildflowers. I know she hasn't been able to tend it lately, but she has always had the energy and shrewdness to improve what she has, and to make the landscape—whether it's a cubicle, a depart-ment, or a yard—homey. And she has had the frugality and patience to wait for 100 free foot0high trees to grow.

I also remember after Charlotte had been in Columbus about two years, she talked about how Christopher and David were forgetting their heritage, that they were beginning to sound Yankee. God forbid! She said very seriously that she was going to have to teach them Virginian so they could continue to talk with the proper accent. And Virginian wasn't just the accent; it included Southern manners, like answering her, "Yes ma'am."

Charlotte is a Southern lady: genteel and soft-spoken, with a backbone and determination made of steel.

Lucie

◆   ◆   ◆

Charlotte was relatively new to Columbus and the Methods engineering. I was her supervisor. As things could go with Charlotte, she and I were in the midst of a disagreement about a project of business process. She was holding to her position as only Charlotte could, when she finally said, "Deb, I try to learn something from everybody..."

Now, here's where I start to think that she's going to say something that will boost my ego, something about how smart I am or how well I manage the area. At least I thought she'd concede and see that I was right about the disagreement.

"...and from you," Charlotte went on, "I want to learn how to dress!"

Over the years, Charlotte and I continued to have our disagreements. We usually respected each other, and ultimately we remained friends. I've learned a lot from Charlotte over the years, but the lessons over the past two-and-a-half years have been the most poignant.

Thank you, Charlotte!

Deb

◆   ◆   ◆

I remember arriving in San Antonio and getting to the hotel just in time to catch Charlotte and some others (Mark Bergstedt and maybe Sharon Manwarren?) headed out to dinner. Dropping luggage to turn around and head out with them, I wasn't involved in on any planning, so I wasn't quite sure what to expect of the after-dinner destination—a hole in the wall along the river Walk called "Dirty Nellie's." True to a

Charlotte form, however, it turned out to be a wonderfully entertaining little pub, and far more respectable than the name implies.

Tim

◆   ◆   ◆

Many memories of Methods Engineering have faded, but one that really stands out for me is the time I was called into a "special meeting" in a conference room. I remember wondering what was going on and whether there was a major problem with our project.

It turned out to be a surprise baby shower for me that Charlotte had secretly put together! I think even my wife Susan was there along with most of Methods. It was a total shock and surprise! It was also a little embarrassing because it was a bit unusual for men to have showers! Also, some of the gifts were not what men usually receive and open in front of people they work with. So as I opened the gifts, it was with "mixed emotions."

In any case, it was a wonderful, thoughtful gesture that I now look back on with many good feelings. The mixed emotions I felt at the time have now become a strong, loving memory of someone who gave of herself to others. She touched my life in a special way.

Dan

◆   ◆   ◆

When I think of Charlotte, I can't isolate one particular memory. More than 15 years of them cascade through my mind in a series of flashes that make up my memory of Charlotte.

The first project Charlotte and I worked on together in Methods Engineering was the feasibility of centralized mail in the fall of 1981. We concluded that it would never work for Nationwide!

The picnic she held at her house for all of Methods—what a glorious, sunny day that was! I remember admiring Charlotte's ability to be so laid back, even with all these people coming, expecting to be entertained. But she really seemed to enjoy herself that day, and so did the rest of us.

One year she told a group of us in Methods that what she wanted for her birthday was a "parasol." A "parasol?" That didn't seem quite in character. It was only after we griller her unrelentingly that she explained it would be easier for her to cut wood if she had a "parasol." Oh, for heaven sakes, Charlotte, of course—a power saw!

And the way she used to run on about "my boys!" Christopher and David hung Charlotte's moon and sky. She was so proud of them and their accomplishments. Everything they did was cause for celebration.

Then there was that black day when I learned she had breast cancer and was taking an extremely aggressive approach to treat it. I think I cried that night.

But there were wonderfully uplifting days, too. Like the one when she called me—I was working at home—to tell me her test results all showed the cancer was receding, and she was NOT going to give up! We both cried on the phone that day. It was the first time she told me, "I love you, Jo." And we never had another conversation that didn't end like that.

The last time I saw Charlotte was in mid-February. Denis (my husband) and I drove up to see her and got to meet Calvin and the boys—boys? I mean those handsome, polite young men they had grown up to be!

Charlotte was in the lounge chair, and while her mind was a lot sharper than mine was, she was feeling physically weak and so tired. "I'm just waiting, Jo, just waiting," she said. "I'm just so tired." I knew—hoped—it wouldn't be long for her.

When Mary called to tell me Charlotte had died, my first though was a selfish one, about how much I'll miss her. But the thought that followed has stuck with me: Charlotte has earned the peace she has today. She is exactly where she wants to be now—although we all know Charlotte won't put up with peace for long. She's probably up there now advising her beloved God on what His next steps should be!

Jo Alice

◆   ◆   ◆

Charlotte and I were new unit supervisors working under Jim Buckalew in Lynchburg. Jim held monthly management meetings off-site. Most of his management team had been around for a long time.

At one of these meetings, Jim was explaining the vacation guidelines and how seniority applies to them, and Charlotte and I disagreed with the policy. As the newest members of the management team, those guidelines just didn't seem fair at all, and we mouthed off about it.

Later, Jim found both of us and thanked us for our honesty in expressing our opinions. Little did he know we just hadn't had enough sense to know when to keep quiet!

Marie

◆   ◆   ◆

One time when we (several folks from Methods engineering and maybe Mary Teter) were in Walnut Creek, California, training on commercial workflows, we decided to go out after work. We ended up at what was probably the only Country & western bar in northern California. We got there a bit early, and it turned out that the establishment was people the Texas Two-Step. Well, guess who I ended up out on the dance floor with—good ol' Charlotte.

Charlotte was reluctant at first—that's right, our headstrong, take-charge, say almost anything Charlotte was hesitant—at least until she eyes a good-looking cowboy on the other side of the room. The she suddenly was very interested in going out on the dance floor. She formulated a plan, and as we stepped out on the dance floor, she explained.

If the good-looking cowboy wanted to cut in while we were dancing, that was OK. I'd allow him to dance with Charlotte, but I had to be sure to work in the fact I was her brother. Charlotte wanted to be sure the guy knew she was "available." Of course, if someone tried to cut in that Charlotte didn't want to dance with, she'd give me a nod, and then I was to be her jealous boyfriend.

It worked! The good-looking cowboy did indeed cut in, and Charlotte made it clear that she was dancing with her "brother," since she didn't know anyone in northern California. I nearly lost it.

John

◆   ◆   ◆

February 25, 1997

Dear Christopher and David,

You may remember the story of your train trip slightly different that I have retold it. That is OK since you were there and I was not.

The train story represents my memory of the impressions that you mother left upon me more so than the family vacation that you shared for which I could never do justice retelling.

Our prayers are with you. God bless you and Charlotte.

Dan

Charlotte's Summer Vacation

Charlotte and her sons prepared to leave for a three-day cross-country train vacation to the American West. Charlotte involved all her coworkers in planning the family vacation, which was only appropriate since Charlotte always treated everyone like family.

Her energy was boundless and her enthusiasm infectious. Everyone contributed ideas.

"Did you say that you were traveling through Denver? You have to stop at this restaurant. It has great food."

"You should get one of those small hairdryers. They save a lot of space and weight."

"Don't forget to pack snacks for the trip. Two boys will bankrupt you buying snacks."

"Do you have lightweight luggage?"

"You have to stop and see Pike's Peak!"

For every suggestion, Charlotte had the same enthusiastic, vigorous response that everyone within a ten-workstation radius could hear, "Thank you. My BOYS will love doing that! Or, my BOYS will need that! Or, my BOYS will really appreciate that!"

There was no denying the unabashed love and affection in her voice for her sons as she pronounced the words, MY BOYS!

It would be easy for a cynical person to think that Charlotte was using her sons to hide the fact she was looking forward to the trip with greater anticipation than her sons. They didn't know Charlotte.

She planned the trip with painstaking detail even to the point of packing the bags with their outfits packed in the same order as they would be needed in different climates. Everyone was going to be happy, healthy, and well dressed for their adventures. All the details were precisely planned.

The big day arrived and the family was caught in the excitement of the hustle and bustle of the train station. There was much to see and hear to absorb the entire experience of their first long distance train trip.

The bags were entrusted to a porter for delivery to the train. Freed form toting numerous bags of luggage, they explored and savored the entire experience. Finally, they received the announcement to board. They checked out the train cars and met many of the employees along the way. As Charlotte proudly led her sons through the corridors, her enthusiastic greetings were usually returned by a smiling employee and the question, "Is this your first train trip?"

The trip was underway before Charlotte, Christopher, and David settled into their sleeping compartment. At first, Charlotte was concerned when the bags were not waiting for them in their sleeping compartment. She was relieved to learn that the bags had been checked and were safely in the baggage compartment.

The good news was quickly forgotten when she heard the attendant's response to her request for him to deliver the bags to their compartment. "I am sorry ma'am, but the luggage cannot be removed from the baggage compartment until we arrive at the final destination."

Their only supplies for the three days were the clothes on their backs and the single package of breath mints in Charlotte's purse.

What a disaster you say! Don't underestimate Charlotte.

The trip became an opportunity for another adventure and a reason to meet people. She traded stories with more passengers during the next three days than during the entire trip. Of course, she told us, her fellow employees and extended family, everyone of those stories with the same passion and excitement as when she first experienced them.

Charlotte frequently referred to the train trip west. It wasn't unusual for someone to ask, "What did you do on the way back?" Charlotte always answered with what they saw and did, but you could tell that the experience was not on the same level as the first trip west.

People were the catalyst that excited Charlotte. That excitement gave her the ability to extract the greatest amount of joy and satisfaction from every situation.

Charlotte gave the world three wonderful blessings: Christopher, David, and love for people.

John

◆   ◆   ◆

When my family moved across town from an apartment to a new house, Charlotte took charge of my kids, drove them to her house, and allowed them to run around in her yard, keeping them out from underfoot. That's the only way we could have moved.

And when our offices moved from Crossroads to Tuttle Crossing, Charlotte was sergeant of that move too. In the weekly meetings she held on the move, almost anytime someone asked about making a change to the floor plan, her response would be, "No changes! No changes!"

Sharon

◆   ◆   ◆

Over 12 years ago I started in the Management Information Systems area of Nationwide Insurance. This was the first time I had supported more the 120 people as their department secretary, including Methods Engineering.

I recall looking forward to the challenge of keeping up with so many professional people. It didn't take long to learn, however, that just because employees have degrees, doesn't mean they are superhuman.

Charlotte stood out among that group of employees. She does possess excellent people skills. It was always a joy to be able to work with Charlotte. It didn't matter if she needed something in a hurry or if it could wait; she always treated me with finesse.

My hope is that someday, when I finally earn my coveted degree, and if secretaries are still members of the team, I will treat my secretary with the same finesse.

Margaret

◆   ◆   ◆

Well all know that Charlotte never lost her southern accent. One day she held a meeting on the floor with the department, as she often did. This meeting was to let us know we were making too many careless errors, but with her accent, it sounded like she was saying, "Guys, we are making too many callous errors."

Well, needless to say, most of us sat dumbfounded because we did not even know that a callous error was, let alone how to begin to clear one.

Then Charlotte realized we did not understand what she was saying, and she kept saying, "Come on guy. You know. Callous errors. You all know what a callous error is." Finally someone said, "Oh, you mean CARELESS error," and we all started laughing, Charlotte included.

Charlotte said, "Yes." That is what I said, callous errors."

Teri

◆   ◆   ◆

One of my favorite memories of Charlotte is a trip I took with her and Ed Chapman to Wausau. We could have taken the company plane and been there in a couple of hours, but Charlotte did not want to fly. So we took a company pool car—a Dodge Dynasty—and headed west for the 13-hour drive.

Charlotte made the trip interesting by pointing out various facts about the places we passed. Ed and Charlotte harassed me often because I need to stop constantly for potty breaks. They made me be quiet for hours before they would stop! At a tollbooth, there was a separate lane for vehicles with three or more axles. Charlotte and Ed tried to make me get out and count the axles on the car so they could leave me there!

When she was not driving, Charlotte worked on a needlepoint tablecloth that she had brought along. She was so into it she forgot how close Ed was and, while pulling the threat through, she stabbed him with the needle. We all got a good laugh out of that.

On the way home, Charlotte made sure that I was dropped off first because she said I whined too much!

Connie

◆   ◆   ◆

In 1984, when Charlotte and I were in Dallas opening the North Texas office, we won a weekend trip to New Orleans. While we were in New Orleans we went on a daytime and a nighttime city tour. We toured up the Mississippi and down the Mississippi on a boat.

We toured the plantations and strolled Bourbon Street. We watched the fireworks being released from a barge out on the Mississippi river, and enjoyed a drink in a revolving restaurant high above the city.

We ate shrimp and crawfish and had beignets and coffee and just had a total blast every minute. Many times we reminisced about this great weekend.

Mary

42

Figuring It Out

When the spring semester was over, I withdrew from OSU. With the passing of Mom, I now had the opportunity to go to film school. There was nothing left in Ohio to keep me from leaving home. David had Dad at home to make sure he finished high school, and there was enough money in the estate to ensure they had everything they needed. The offer at the studio in Orlando was still good; there was nothing in my way this time.

I quit my job at Nationwide and re-enrolled in film school in June. I went to Orlando for a couple of days just to make sure everything was in order. I had been looking forward to this for several years, and it was finally within reach. Everything I had been reaching towards for so long was in sight, but the insecurity of life had shaken the unrelenting confidence I once had.

When Mom died, half of my family died with her. David was the only blood relative left that had endured everything life brought into my family. Dad had been around, but he was a weekend dad. In my late teens his visits had become less and less as I grew into adulthood. He was a visitor, not the constant in my home. Mom had been the reassuring security for both my brother and I throughout our lives. She had been the one to catch us before we fell or to help us get back up. With her gone, the safety net I always counted on was gone.

If I fell, I would not have anyone reaching down to help pull myself back up. While in Florida, the loss of this security wove its way into my thoughts and slowly drained the confidence I had just a few months before. The world suddenly looked far more dangerous than it had previously, and for the first time, I put on hold what I wanted more than anything in world.

I decided to hold off on film school for a year. David would be starting his senior year in high school, and I knew Dad and him did not get along. I used David as an excuse to back out of the uncertainty. Instead of overcoming obstacles in the way of becoming a director/producer, I created the road blocks to justify my own insecurities about life. This hesitation would become an unraveling decision that would eventually lead to many self inflicted problems.

When I returned to Ohio, the dreams of film school left in Florida, I did whatever I could to keep myself active. Instead of returning to school, I went into real estate sales and investing. I put the money I had set aside for film school into investment property with the intention of selling the property when I finally made the choice to go back to school. Like many people, I put many things aside in my life figuring I would have plenty of time and plenty of opportunities to pick up where I left off.

I did very well with my real estate studies, passed the examinations required for licensing at the top of my class, and moved through life with the lingering enthusiasm left over after making a choice to wait a year before following that for which I truly had a passion.

Almost immediately, I knew staying was a mistake. It would be a couple of years before I would realize how significant the mistake was, but regret began sinking in right away. I no longer had the desire to get to work early and work late. I no longer pursued dancing or the theater. I just wanted to do what I needed to do to get by and go home. The essence of the life experience had been lost to me.

To add to this, it was thought having Dad stay with us would be a good idea. David is just under two years younger than myself and was still in high school. The thought behind him moving in was to ensure David stayed out of trouble and to lend fatherly assistance, but it turned out just the opposite. Both David and I had dealt with Dad in the past and had had problems with him before, but figured this would be the opportunity we would need to reconcile the differences, but those differences would just grow over the next couple of years.

I quickly found out, having someone visit every once in a while, or visiting them over summer vacation was far different than living with that person. Dad mixed with us like oil mixing with water, especially when it came to David and Dad getting along. I had the constant job of mediating fights and solving childish problems between the two on a regular basis. Every night there was something new brooding between the two of them turning my childhood home into a den of strife with apprehension just beneath the surface.

By my own volition, I made two wrong decisions and paid severely for many years to follow. I can look back on my life and see many of my problems started just months after my mother's death—not directly because of the loss, but because of how I reacted to the loss. When I took the step not to go to school and to invite Dad into ours lives, I did not see the consequences of that fork in my life. I can not tell anyone what would have happened if I had went to Florida instead of staying in Ohio, I just know I messed up and continued to choose unwisely. Once I started on the path, it was an easy ride to the bottom.

Life for the next several years would be a downward spiral for me, my brother, and my dad. Even though there were many who repeatedly warned me of the dangerous road I was skipping down, nothing would be able to get in my way of self-destruction. I would have to see the harsh reality of the end before I would turn around and claw my way back up.

PART IV
Self Destruction

43

Bad Ideas, Bad Choices

Everyone looks back on their life and wishes they could go back and change the mistakes they have made throughout the years. I should have never come back to Ohio when I was standing at the doorstep of film school, but I chose another road. It is curious to look back, knowing what I know, seeing those paths in my life and realizing how similar they were. Staying in Ohio for a few years or jumping into a new school both seemed good ideas.

Making a bad choice most often looks like a good idea or the right way to go. I was knee deep in a tangled web of bad choices before I even knew what I was standing in. I was knotted up before I even realized life was tying me down. After I started, it was easy to continue to make decisions that would only speed up the downward trend. Eventually, I started to make even worse choices to cover up or correct the bad choices. The snowball had started in my life, and it was determined to grow larger and larger until it finally hit the rock wall at the bottom of the hill.

Becoming a real estate agent in Centerburg was just the first step into the hole that would eventually become my life. I became an agent to get out of the house. Dad was driving me crazy, and David and he fought constantly. Being a real estate agent lacked a stern overhead authority—something I desperately needed at the time. I was not required to be in the office at any given time. There were not many expectations placed on me. I could do what I wanted when I wanted.

I used my real estate agent status as a way to get away when it suited me. I did not have the desire to work. Not that I was lazy, I was just not content with what I wanted to be doing. I went into the real estate office regretting not pursuing my film aspirations. Eventually, I went into the office with the expectation I would be leaving soon and that I was just biding my time.

Just a few months earlier, I was studying most of my nights to do well in school. I had to keep a solid GPA to retain my scholarships for film school. I went to work early and did everything I could to retain a great reference for the studio I would be working for in Florida. Everything was geared to the dreams I was striving to achieve. Now, time had just become something that must run by. I had walked away from the past hopes of my future and had not replaced them with new hopes. Life was just a routine for me, and it had only taken two months. Years had been spent planning and looking ahead, but in a simple whiff it was gone.

Even though it was a complete failure, all was not lost in my real estate endeavors. I met some of the best people Centerburg and the Knox county community has to offer. Bob, who was the main agent in the Centerburg office, is one of the best sales professionals I have met. He is one of the most charismatic and genuine person I have had the pleasure of working with. No matter how bad things became in my life, and I am sure he was aware of the many problems I was having, he never looked down on me or made me feel like a less of a person because of my failures.

I will always remember him, not so much for his selling skills, but for having lunch with me and not throwing the mistakes I had made at me. The world would be a better place if we had fewer judgmental people and more like Bob. Most people know what they have done wrong. Most people will deal with their problems themselves. They just need someone to have lunch with every once in a while and not constantly be reminded of the problems riding their backs.

It did not take to long before I started out on yet another venture to help settle my restlessness. I went back into the business I knew through my mother and the part time job while in college at Ohio State. I stepped back into the insurance field, but this time, instead of claims, I was on the other end of the spectrum—sales. I should have learned from the real estate blunders that sales was not something I was going to be succeeding with. It is not that I can not do sales; I was just in a mind set to do what I needed to do to just pass time. I was not really interested in selling anything, or putting in the work to grow a successful sales base. But again, I stepped into something just to be doing something different, just to kill more time, all the while digging a deeper hole for myself.

I started out working for the local Nationwide agent. Donna set me up with an office and gave me the ability to write insurance policies and set me loose. My office was in a renovated house that was shared with an attorney. Jim had been the attorney who handled the final requests of my mother, so he was a familiar face, and we became pretty good friends while I was there.

Like real estate, insurance sales was exciting for a couple of weeks. The hole was still there in my life and this had not filled it or resolved my ravenous discontentment with life. Soon I began showing up to work like I had at the real estate office. I came in to work as an opportunity to get away from home or to pass the days as they ticked away leading to nothing particular.

I ended up spending more time talking with Jim's secretary than actually doing work. I spent many hours surfing the internet, searching but finding nothing. I would do a little work if someone called in for a quote, and I looked professional when someone came in off the street, but most of my time was spent waiting. I was snoozing in life's waiting room anticipating the moment when life would call my name.

I had to be behind my desk for most of the day while I was pretending to be an insurance agent. When I was doing real estate, I could come and go as I pleased. I did not have the responsibility of opening the doors in the morning or closing up at night. Now I had set hours. That left a lot of time for me to do nothing, and to think about how bad life was getting.

David and I were spending money by the buckets. We were spending a great deal more than we were bringing in, never minding the bottom was in sight. David was spending money to do mindless activities with his friends. I was spending money to give myself value to those around. I bought computers, cars, houses, everything I could get my hands on. We were spending the money our mother had left us like it had no end. We did not realize it had taken her years to acquire what she had, and we were blowing it faster than the receipt machines could spit out the sales tickets.

David was looking for a place to fit in. His home life had been destroyed with Mom's death, and Dad was only making things worse. I was looking for a reason to justify the stupid choice I had made with school. Both of us sought something we would never find in the places we went, the people we knew, or the things we bought. But we did not see it then. We had hope the next day would bring back something of the past.

I sat in that insurance office day after day, doing nothing but waiting and watching. With all the free time I had created for myself due to my lack of motivation, I started the novel *The Xebec*. At the time, it was untitled, but it gave me a non-judgmental way of looking at my situation. The characters took on the personalities of those around me and even myself. Like everything I had written in the past, this story reflected a part of my life that I never thought I would see. I was loosing the hope of tomorrow due to the mistakes of the past, and things still would get far worse before they ever began to get better.

Almost before I had completely unpacked, I was on the move again. This time I was going out completely on my own. I started my own insurance agency with just a few backing insurance companies and left everyone behind. I used this opportunity to isolate myself from those around me. I did not want to start my own business; I just needed a place to go. I just needed a place that I could consider my own.

I would have thought I would have been level headed enough to see I was trotting right into the abyss. The real estate escape had failed; the insurance escape had failed; everything was going to fail until I changed, but I went forward. I had not learned my lesson. I had poured thousands of dollars into the past two ventures but was willing to do it again just to start something new. Thousands of dollars were spent just for something to do.

Just like yesterday, the money I had needed for school was now gone and there would be nothing I could do to ever get it back. More importantly, I had lost my drive to go to school. Even if the money was not gone, I would not have been able follow the dreams of the past.

I had radically changed direction three times in two years, spent countless thousands trying to fill a hole, but I had to stay away from home whenever possible. Almost running parallel with my career and financial situation, my home life was running itself into the ground. I would do anything not to have to go home in the evenings. I would watch television late into the night at my new insurance agency, just to avoid going home.

44

Dissension Enters the Home

It is hard to really appreciate what a person does or means to you when they are still around. During their absence one learns and develops a respect for what the omitted person in their life meant to them. A husband always appreciates what his wife does when she goes away for a weekend—gains an understanding of her contribution to his family. A child longs for his mother when she leaves Dad to care for the house.

I did not see what my mother had done for me until she was gone. The house I called home was always clean and filled with food when she was alive. Problems I considered insurmountable were resolved when she was around. Fights between David and I were mediated when she was alive, and Dad was brought into the family when she was alive. I was about to learn what can happen to a person when just one person in their life is missing.

Dad had now come into our lives full time. He had decided to move into the home that had been complete with David, myself, and mom. He was a stranger who now wanted to play Dad to two sons he only saw on holidays and monthly visits. He walked through our door as if he owned the place.

All three of us were looking for something, and living in a house were every-one is looking to fill a void will lead to dissonance among everyone in the house-hold. I was wondering if I should have stayed in Florida. David was looking for a future—unsure about anything the world had to offer, and Dad was looking for the family he had lost many years ago.

We were like every other person in world looking towards others to make their lives whole or to find happiness. David was looking towards me for direc-tion—something I was lacking completely. Dad was looking to recapture the years past with his sons—something he could never get back from us, and I was looking for reassurance from a dad who could not provide it.

As time went by, all of us had to face the hard reality; the answers to our ques-tions and our pursuits of happiness would not be found within each other. David and Dad fought constantly over the most mundane and petty instances, catching me in the middle to referee fights that could not be won or lost on either side. They just got under each other's skin in such a way that prevented them from ever being in the same room for more than a few moments.

David chose the company of his friends over that of his family and did everything to avoid even being seen with Dad. Dad sought the bottle in order to drown out his failures, and I stayed at a deteriorating insurance agency just to be away from them both. Regardless of my ineptness as a sales professional, I was grateful for a place to go. I was paying rent, utilities, and keeping up the appearance of working a business just to avoid the problems at home. Before I had been going into the office for something to do, but I soon went in to get away from the realities of home and the looming self-inflicted problems rising just over the horizon.

My childhood home had become a place of ruin and filth. Anyone who had visited my mother before her death would have seen a house that was well kept, a yard that was well trimmed, and felt a peace within its walls. With the three of us left, the yard was quickly filled with car parts Dad had started carting in from every junkyard in Ohio. The yard grew out of control, and the interior began to pile up with the grime of three men living under one roof—none of us having a desire to care for that for which we had.

When one of us did take an interest in something at the house, the others seemed to undue that interest every time. David would clean up the yard only to have Dad fill it with rusted car parts or complete junked cars. I would vacuum and dust only to come home to a vomit filled carpet from over drinking by Dad. Dad would clean the dishes in the house to have David and his friends come over and dirty them all up just hours after they were cleaned—not making an effort to clean them themselves.

We had become our own worse enemies. At a time when we needed each other the most, we did everything possible to avoid the others and everything we could to distress each other. There was never any compromise, just conflict. Each of us blamed the others for our failures and never looked to one another for solutions, just scapegoats.

Mirroring everything else in my life, the house started to fall apart. Holes started to appear in the walls from fights. The carpeting began to show large spots from oily car parts and spilt drinks from sloppy and often tipsy quests. Empty beer bottles and cans rattled throughout the house as Dad went from bottle to bottle with no end in sight. Ashtrays overflowed; the sink was bursting with dirty dishes; the refrigerator housed more mold than food; the bathroom floor was gritty with dirt, and dust coated everything, giving the house a dingy gray tint.

Everything had gone wrong. I no longer was pursuing a college education. I was quickly digging a very deep financial hole. The house I had grown up in had gone from a charming country home to a fixer upper, and I was distancing myself from the remaining family left in my life.

In just under two years, I went from a life filled with a struggle to achieve to a struggle to resolve unrelenting troubles. I was not taking steps forward or even maintaining my current position in life. I was fighting to prevent myself from being thrown off the staircase of life all together. Everything in my life had broken or was in the process of breaking and no effort on my part could stop what I had set into motion.

Nothing could stop what I had created from my simple lack of enthusiasm for life and what the future held for me and for those around me. Just by not caring, I had opened a door to the pit that would swallow everything around me. I used to think the notion of failure at life was worse then stepping out on the limb, but I soon realized not doing anything was just as bad, if not worse, than doing something wrong. At least if I had taken my chances with past dreams, I had chance of making something of myself, but by sitting aside idol waiting for something to happen I had unknowingly stepped into the failure I feared, which prevented me from going to Florida.

Soon the disposable funds dried up. Bills were being paid late. Only minimum payments were being sent into creditors, and the quick fix of material possessions came to a halt with a mailbox filled with overdue accounts. I have found it to be a good assumption that everything seems to happen in threes. I had lost my confidence and was killing time looking busy but going nowhere. My home life became unrecognizable, and now I was broke. I had my three strikes—all my doing, all brought on by the choices I had made.

Anyone who has ever lived apart from million dollar trust funds, know financial problems can cause some of the most devastating blows to a person's life. Marriages have been broken, families separated, self-esteem crushed, and friendships lost, all over the mismanagement of money. Money is a bondage that holds tighter than illness, family discord, tragic loss, and anything else life has to throw at a person, and it had its noose around my neck.

Many people had warned me, but there is no one deafer than someone who will not listen. I only listen when the threat of loosing my home was a real possibility. It took the fear of not having a place to live for me to light a fire under myself and see the reality of the situation I was facing, the incredible blunders, and to make a decision to at least not go any further into the abyss. I now had to save whatever I could before it went down the drain. I know longer had the luxury of going to work for the sole purpose of getting away from home. I no longer had the time, to think about what I wanted to do. It was time to do something or loose everything.

45

Just What Needed to Be Done

Sometimes deciding what to keep is harder than deciding what to seek. I had to look over everything in my life and decide what I wanted to fight for—what I thought was worth keeping and what should be let go. Following the pattern of the previous two years, I choose to do only what I needed to do to keep my head afloat. Everything else was dispensable.

Within just weeks of receiving final notice for the mortgage on my childhood home, I closed my playhouse insurance agency and went to work. I ended up at a small insurance company in Columbus providing customer service to policyholders. Again, I found myself working in an industry I had no desire to be in but that was all I knew. The time to step into something new had passed. What I knew was insurance; and it would be the only way I would have to prevent further loss.

Even with my continued attitude of only doing what was necessary to prevent further loss, the challenge of saving what was left brought my dad, David, and I closer. We had a common goal, something all of us wanted but never could find between the three of us until collection companies started to knock at our door. These problems were something that affected us all and would take the efforts of all of us to resolve them. We were not able to build a bond between the three of us, but we were able to work together to resolve common problems. It was exactly what was needed, but we all wished we had found another way.

Within just a couple of months of David and I working, we started to see some results. Even though these results were tenuous at best, both of us started to see we could make a difference on the world in which we lived. We both saw that hard work does lead to accomplishments.

As time continued to go by, I found myself not working to just save what needed to be saved, but also to dig myself out of the hole I had dug for myself. For once, life was a tangible objective. There was a reason to work instead of just killing time until something better came along.

Dad was able to mesh himself into his two son's lives. He finally had a part of what went on and became a part of the solution instead of a part of the problem. Arguments occurred less and less and our home eventually turned into a refuge from the world similar to what it had once been. It never completely returned to what it once was; we were more like three people working together to achieve a common objective, but never really getting to know one another or to allow the others into our individual personal worlds. During the day we played nice together but went our separate ways at night. But even this thin thread of civility between the three of us was better than the chaos and strife of the past.

When Thanksgiving finally rolled around, the three of us had been able to stabilize our lives enough to maintain our standard of living. With this Thanksgiving being the first of the new millennium, life was starting to brighten a bit. This first year was not only the start of a new century, but it was a new start to our lives. I had created many problems for myself, but I had them under control and was working my way to a better future. It would never be like I had imagined years before, but at least I could see some light at the end instead of the bottom getting closer by each passing day.

For the last several years I had dreaded the holiday seasons. Mom had been the one to make Thanksgiving and Christmas magical for the family. With her gone, I just assume skip over the holidays and drown them out with work or some mindless activity that would suppress the memories of the past, but I was looking forward to this Thanksgiving. I had been working long hours and putting everything I had into saving as much as I could of my life. All the hard work, sleepless nights, and struggling had paid off. Things were starting to stabilize, and I looked forward to a few days off.

I had lucked out this holiday weekend. David would be spending it with friends, and Dad was going to Virginia for the holiday. I had the entire place to myself. I did not have the large turkey dinner, but I had a house that was quiet. Never had silence been so comforting and relaxing. I may not have had anyone around, but I was content and savored every moment. Still had a lot to do and I did not know when I would get the opportunity to read a book without interruption, watch television in silence, and be able to take an afternoon nap. After the holiday, it would be back to the task of correcting the daunting troubles I had created.

46

It Visits Again

It had just been three years since my mother had lost her battle with cancer. In that time I had managed to ruin most of the opportunities I had before her death. I had self destructed everything she had left to my brother and I, and I was struggling just to get from one day to the next. I had turned into the person I feared. I had failed at everything I had done since her death, and I was now going through life doing what I had to do just to survive. I used to work and go to school to do what I loved, but I had now turned into everyone else. Life had pressed in on me so hard due to my loss of motivation; I had to fight for every breath I took. I never meant for this happen. I wanted to be someone who lived life always reaching for something better, but I was now settling for anything that would pay the bills and put food on the table.

After the Thanksgiving holiday, David came home to get ready to head back out into the weeks ahead filled with long days and very little gratification for all the hard work. Dad returned from Virginia with news that would again strain an already squeezed household.

Since Dad was on total disability for his injuries from Vietnam, he was required to have regular checkups at a Veterans hospital in order to maintain his status. When he went to Virginia for Thanksgiving, he stopped by the Veterans hospital in Salem, Virginia. Not quite being accustomed to the cold of Ohio's falls and winters, he had a hard time fighting off the flu. His sinuses swelled and the glands in his neck inflated as they tried to rid his body of infection.

He asked his doctor for some antibiotics for the infection that would not seem to go down in his neck. The nightly doses of NyQuil and Tylenol were not getting the job done. He felt well, but the knot in his neck would not go down this time as it had in the past. It throbbed just behind his left ear and in the back of his throat. The doctor did some tests, drew some blood, and wrote out a prescription for some drugs to make the swelling go down.

Being in a hurry to leave, Dad asked the doctor for a couple of doses, instead of waiting for the prescription to be filled at the hospital pharmacy. A friend and him were going to the Florida Keys for the holiday instead of spending it in the cold mountains of Virginia. Already knowing it would take an hour or so for the pharmacy to get him his medication, he just needed enough to last a few days so he could get on his way to Florida. On his trip back through to Ohio, he would stop by and pick up the full doses.

The doctor agreed, not really even sure if the flu was the reason for the swelling, and gave him enough to last the holiday season. Instead of going to the pharmacy to pick up the prescription, the doctor asked that my dad stop by his office after the holiday. He would have the drugs he needed, and all the tests back by the time Dad returned. The doctor wanted to make sure he was prescribing the right medication for my dad's ailments.

After a weekend in the sun and hanging out on the beach with his friends, Dad returned to his doctor's office to get his medication. The doctor told him he did not need antibiotics, but instead, needed aggressive throat and neck surgery, months of chemotherapy, and multiple radiation treatments. The lump he had in the side of his neck and throat was actually a cancer tumor caused by excessive drinking and years of smoking. He had probably had the tumor for a while, but it had grown to the size of a soft ball and was just starting to cause a good deal of pain when he moved his head.

Out in his shop, the day after he returned from his holiday adventures, Dad told me what the doctor had said. This time when he spoke of his medical conditions, he was not doing so for attention or for the pity of others. This time the only thing in his eyes was fear. For years he had been telling everyone who would listen how bad his health was deteriorating. Now he wished he could tell me everything was alright, that he was healthy.

I asked what he was going to do. Both of us knew first hand what radiation, chemotherapy, and surgery meant. It was not that long ago that we had been through it with Mom. He told me, he had to be in Salem, Virginia, after the first of the year to begin his long road to the end. Sometimes I think Dad died that afternoon when the doctor told him what was growing in his neck. He was now just going through the motions because the doctors said he ought to do so, but not because he was willing to fight.

David and I reassured him we were there for him. We may not have always seen eye to eye nor had the best relationships in the past, but that was all behind us. Dad was the last parent we had. He may not have always done the right things, but he always had the best of intentions. He had stood with David and I through Mom's death and was doing everything he could to help the two of us find our ways or at least stay standing while we found our places.

Unlike the tenuous bond that had been formed between the three of us as we worked to correct the deficiencies in our lives, the hardships Dad was facing would bring David and I close together and hopefully build the needed bond between us and our dad. I had been working overtime hours, without vacation and sick leave, and had some savings and plenty of paid time off from work. This would give me the opportunity to be with Dad as he started his crossing.

That Christmas and New Year holiday was filled with the dread of the coming year. We had just started to turn ourselves around when life had dealt us a blow none of us were ready to bare. David and I had loads of support through our mother's battle with cancer and eventual death, but this time, everything would by on our shoulders. I looked ahead and saw a predetermined road that I did not want to take. I was not ready for what lay ahead but was going to be forced to face it head on.

After the first of the year, Dad and I drove to Virginia to prepare for the first rounds of surgery that would begin his cancer treatment. David had to wait a few weeks before he could get some time off from work, but would be joining the two of us shortly. The day before the surgery Dad had to check into the hospital to get his blood work done and for an extensive checkup.

That night I did not sleep much. I was staying with a friend of Dad's in Lynchburg, but felt completely alone. Even though my blood family was all around, I desired the comfort and company of my friends in Ohio. These people were strangers to me.

With the restless night behind me, I was back in Salem by four AM the next morning. Dad was scheduled to go into surgery at five and I wanted to be there before they took him away. I was able to get there in time to have the hospital breakfast and talk to him for a few minutes. When the time came, both of us walked the long corridors of the old hospital to the surgical ward. The conversation we had during that walk would be the last time I would ever hear his voice, and it would be the last time he ever looked like the dad of my past.

After dragging our feet for as long as we could, we made it to the oncologist ward of the hospital, and he was taken right in; I was directed to the waiting room to sit and imagine worst case scenarios for the next several hours. This room filled with uncomfortable chairs, stark white walls, florescent lights, and year old magazines would be my frustrating world while I waited.

After an hour of pacing, I went to the gift shop and bought some pens and paper. To help me forget my worries, I began to write. Writing had always been the one place I could go where my problems did not follow. During the long hours spent waiting, I wrote *Rich Hill*. *Rich Hill* gave me the strength to sit and let time pass. It gave me the opportunity to put into words everything that had transpired the last couple of years within the fabric of a horrific tale of ancient powers lurking just under the surface of Centerburg's sweet fields of corn and soy.

Eventually, trying to take care of my obligations in Ohio and be by my father's side was starting to run me haggard. I could not continue being in both places. David and I were running on fumes forcing us to make a decision as to what to do next. We could not be in Ohio and Virginia at the same time. We had to choose where we were going to focus our efforts. Another critical crossroad had presented itself to us and our decision either way would affect everything in our lives.

47

Lynchburg

Our decision to move to Virginia was a very hard one to make. Everything David and I knew was in Ohio. Our friends were there; our jobs were there; and the familiarity of Centerburg was there. Leaving, meant leaving everything we knew at a time in our lives when we needed familiar surrounding to reassure us life would be alright for the two of us.

The only up side to leaving was its resolve to many of our problems. By selling everything out, we would clear ourselves of the debts we had incurred and be given the opportunity to start over in a new city, in a new house, with new jobs. The constant reminders of our shortcomings over the last few years could be left behind for the hopes of a better tomorrow. The memories of the past could finally be put in the past. We could start fresh.

In April of 2001, David and I moved into a new house in Lynchburg, Virginia, leaving behind our lives in Ohio to help our ill father and to start something completely new. We took everything that was dear to us and left the heartache of the last three years behind.

Everything was going well the first several months. Dad was still in the hospital undergoing treatments, and David and I were settling into our new home. I picked up a job at a local catalog retailer, and David found work at the local home improvement center. For once in a long time, bills were getting paid, our home life was peaceful, and each day was not filled with the constant worries of survival.

Every other day, David and I would make the hour long trip to the hospital to check up on Dad and enquire about his progress. As the days turned into weeks, the weeks into months, we started to see our dad return to a resemblance of the man he once was. The scars behind his ear and down his neck were starting to heal, and the sight of him missing half the flesh on the left side of his neck was becoming less and less shocking to the two of us. The hole left in the middle of his throat for breathing became something we could handle, along with the feeding tube hanging from his stomach.

David and I were dealing with something I had had doubts we would ever have been able to handle on our own. We were meeting new people each day at work, and we had everything ready at the house for Dad when he finally was released from the hospital. We had made it through the many hospital trips watching our dad wither away. We had made it through the move to a new state, and we were ready for Dad when he came home. Having a sick person in our home was nothing new to David and I.

I do not know when David started to question the move to Virginia, but I do know when I did. In June as I was going to Salem to bring home my dad, it hit me that what I had done was irreversible. I would not be able to go home for a very long time. David and I had let everything go in order to be close to our dad in his time of need. By doing this, we were able to get a nice house in Lynchburg, but we had also closed the door to returning. Neither of us had the resources to back out of this decision.

The night before I had finished *Rich Hill* and placed the four notebooks into the box in the attic that contained the other stories I had written over the years about my home town. When I closed the lid, I closed the lid on Centerburg and everything that town and its people had meant to me. As I drove, I could only hope I had made a better choice than I had years before when I returned to Ohio from Florida. Had I taken the easy way out by moving? Should I have stayed in Ohio and fought for what was mine instead of giving it all up? Hoping that I had done the right thing was all I had left

48

Rock Bottom Closes In

Before Dad ever came home from the hospital, David and I had spent many long hours getting our new home into order. We made sure everything was in its place so he would not have to worry with any of the details. The supplies he would need to care for himself were bought and stored. A bedroom with all the essentials and comforts was setup for him. The first day after his release, all he had to do was get the rest he needed.

I had dealt with Mom when she was sick, and I understood the messes a sick person makes. The problems they have getting around, and the mood swings they have because of the constant pain. Both, David and I, were ready for the long weeks ahead of us, but we made the mistake of going about caring for Dad similar to the care we had given our mother. He would prove to be a very different home patient than our mother had been and cause us some of the greatest emotional pains either of us had ever had to endure.

Everything Dad did seemed to be to give David and I grief. We understood he was sick, but he never once would do anything to help us as we tried to care for him. He would vomit wherever he was standing; never even attempting to make it to the bathroom or the trashcans we kept in his bedroom and bedside the sofa in the living room. He would just spray the milky contents of his stomach on the walls, on the furniture, or on the floors, anywhere he was when the urge occurred.

Vomit was something I could deal with. He was still not eating through his mouth. He was using his feeding tube to inject Ensure and vitamins directly into his stomach. Consequently, his vomit was similar to milk and easy to clean up, but it was a hassle cleaning the walls and constantly scrubbing the carpet. The chunks of bloody flesh were the things that made me gag.

Dad's throat had not completely healed by the time he was released, and the hole in his throat was still bleeding and had to be kept clean, but Dad would never do it. He would walk around the house with the hole in his throat, crusted over and bloody. When he would cough or heave, pieces of flesh would fling out.

Instead of putting his hand over the hole to catch the chucks he was hacking up, he would allow them to blow out into the room.

In just a few weeks, David and I had to regularly go through the house with a putty knife to scrape the mucus, dried flesh, and blood stains off the walls and ceilings. Every time Dad would use the bathroom, he would come leaving large scabs splattered on the mirror and walls. David and I were not asking for much from him; we just needed a little help keeping things clean. Coming home each night to a house with flesh hanging from the ceiling, running down the walls, and vomit caked into the carpet began to wear on the two of us.

It eventually got so bad, neither David nor I eat in the house. Everywhere we looked, we saw nasty refuse from our Dad. We were doing all we could to keep up with his mess, but it was like he was flinging his scabs throughout the house just to spite David and I—just to see us gag as we cleaned up the mess.

When he figured out he could pour vodka into his feeding tube, we not only had to deal with the retching mess he was creating, but we also had to deal with a drunk father who did not respect himself much less his two sons. We starting coming home from work, finding all kinds of sordid messes in the house and him laying pasted out naked in the backyard or at the kitchen table or some other debauched location. We would have to wrestle him to his room and then spend a couple hours cleaning the mess, just to start over the next day.

The few friends I was making at work were never able to stop by to hang out or play video games. As much as I had tried, I could not get the sour stench of vomit out of the house and was unable to scrape up every piece of flesh on the walls, and I never knew what Dad would be doing. Often he would walk around drunk in a t-shirt bloody from wound around his feeding tube and encrusted with dried boogers and bloody mucus from the hole in his throat. I would ask him to shower and change, even offered to help him if he needed it, but he never did. I could not expose the few people I knew to him, not because I was ashamed of him, but because I did not want to have to clean up their vomit after they saw him.

During the many visits to the hospital, I begged for some help from the doctors. I told them he was drinking through his feeding tube, he would not care for himself the way he should, and he was tormenting both David and I. The doctors told me his cancer was in complete remission. He would be alright once the scars healed and that the hospice services they had were just for terminal patients.

Everything Dad was doing was of his own choice not because he was dying and acting out. His strength was coming back along with his hair, and he had many more years ahead of him. He would never be able to talk again, but his life had been spared. Everything David and I did to get him to lighten up on the messes was returned with nastier, more creative forms of filth. Eventually, we just stopped. We stopped cleaning his room, made him stay out of the kitchen when we were in there and did whatever we could not to go home.

I was right back were I had started. I could no longer go home and did everything I could to stay away. I could no longer deal with a drunken father, a father who seemed to like watching me retch as I cleaned his mess and laughed as I did. Living in that house with my dad and brother was worse then working long hours in Ohio. It was worse then not knowing what to do with my life or where I should be going. It was worse than loosing my mother. Not only did I have to deal with a disrespectful, unruly father, but I was all alone. I had left everyone of importance to me, other than David, in Ohio.

The end was close. I had staved off rock bottom in Ohio by working hard, but had only sped things up by moving to Lynchburg. This time, there would not be a way out until I hit the very bottom.

49

We Were Not Worth It

With Dad being so horrible to David and I, we stayed away from the house as much as possible. We would hang out with friends, spend time with our girl-friends, and even work extra hours just to stay away from home. Additional work, even though tired from a full day's work, was better than going home.

On March 7th 2002, Dad asked me to take him to the store instead of going to work. He was able to drive and had plenty of friends to take him if he did not want to go alone. I was not going out with him looking the way he did in his bloody t-shirt and grimy sweat pants. Without listing to him any further, I left the house. He was already drunk, and I was not in the mood to deal with him the afternoon. My sympathy for him was gone. I could not deal with him purposely spitting up in the store to watch me clean it up.

That night I got home around eleven-thirty. David had already come home from work and was already cleaning up the mess, a nightly routine for the two of us. I helped him finish up so he could go out with his girlfriend for dinner. We still were not able to eat in the house. There were still too many reminders of Dad stuck to the walls. I had eaten before coming home and was in for the night.

Before I took my shower, I peeked into Dad's room to make sure he was not passed out in his chair or on the floor as he so often was. If I left him on the floor or sitting up in his chair, he would wake up with stiff muscles and take his dis-comfort out on David and I. It was easier to just haul him into bed rather than fight with his the next morning.

When I looked in, he was in his chair passed out. I reach over to shake his arm. If I could wake him up enough to him get into bed, I would not have to pick him up. I had just touched his arm for a couple seconds and knew. I looked around to see if I was right. I saw the feeding tube and the four empty bottles of liquor on the floor. Dad had put so much alcohol into his system, he had simply fallen asleep never to wake up again.

My dad lay slumped over in his chair dead. When the paramedics came to remove him, they told me he had been dead for several hours, almost right after I had left for work. He had given up on David and I. For some reason, he felt life with his two sons was worse then dying. Since the cancer had not done it for him, he used Ever Clear. I do not know what I did to him for him to think death was better than life, but whatever it was, I am truly sorry. I look back and wish things could have ended better between the two of us.

I will not forget finding him that night and having to tell David that our dad had died. I had had to tell him Mom had died and did not like giving him this news. His death meant the very end for David and I. The people we had once been died with him that night. Nothing of our former selves was left. We became orphans in a world that was already strangling the life from us.

At the funeral, I watched as people came to pay their respects. I stood by the casket having to be introduced to the people who would say they were family. Unlike Mom's funeral, I had no friends or family present. There were people there who were related to David and I by blood, but none of them were family. The closest thing I had to loved ones present that night were a couple of David's friends from Ohio. None of them were really my friends, but it was great to see some faces from the past. They were the only connection I had to those who really mattered to me.

All I could remember after burying my dad was sickness and death. I tried to remember the good times of my youth, but I could only remember cleaning vomit, hearing cries of pain at night, and death. Since I was seventeen that was all I had to look forward to. Cancer, and everything that comes with the disease, had been with me so long it was all I could remember.

◆   ◆   ◆

The rest of my life lay ahead of me now. David is the only thing I have left, and I can only imagine what will happen next. I would say my outlook on life is good, but every time I look for the positive, tragedy finds its way in.

I have made so many grievous mistakes, I am not sure if I will ever get out from under the thumb of oppression I have allowed to press down on me. At the age of twenty-five, I have cared for two cancer riddled parents, buried them both, ruined many opportunities, and sunk myself into a financial hole so deep I can not even see the light.

I do not know what lies ahead, but it can not be any worse than what has already happened.

Epilog

Since my father's death, I was able to recapture some of the fire to be a horror novelist after finding several stories in my attic. I managed to claw my way out of financial ruin. I have successfully finished my undergraduate degree, completed a Masters of Business Administration and am currently in film school.

It took loosing everything before I had the confidence to strive for something great. It is amazing how having nothing to loose leads to all kinds of opportunities. I sometimes wonder what any of us would be doing if we knew we could not fail. I have moved forward because failure had lost its grip on my life.

David is currently finishing his undergraduate studies and is looking forward to receiving his Masters in Criminal Justice. Both of us have done more in the last few years than we have done in our entire lives. *The Average American Son* is just a portion of my life. I think it is the boring part of my life. It was not until after Dad's death that life really became interesting for the two of us. I look forward to writing the conclusion to this book twenty-five years from now. I can only hope it will be as rich as my first twenty-five years.

David and I have both put the past in the past and are once again moving forward like we had been many years ago. Our horizons are bright with opportunity, and the both of us look forward to what the future holds, instead of dreading what the next year will bring. I finally understand everyone is flawed in some way, has made mistakes in their past, has wasted opportunities, and is looking for direction, but these discrepancies are a part of life everyone must endure in some way. It is the only way we can move forward with life.

Failure, tragedy, and misfortune are simply ends to a flawed past and the beginnings of a new start, something all of us need throughout life.

0-595-34282-5

www.ingramcontent.com/pod-product-compliance
Lightning Source LLC
Chambersburg PA
CBHW061348280526
45784CB00001B/176